BULLETPROOF
DIET

*Weight Loss, More Energy and Better
Focus with the Bulletproof Diet*

BONUS! OVER 60+ BULLETPROOF
DIET RECIPES FOR BEGINNERS!

VALERIE CHILDS

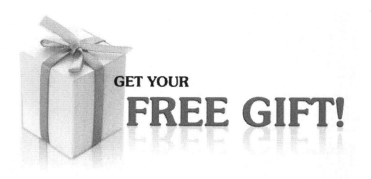

GET YOUR

FREE GIFT!

WAIT! – DO YOU LIKE FREE BOOKS?

My **FREE Gift** to You!! As a way to say **Thank You** for downloading my book, I'd like to offer you more **FREE BOOKS!** Each time we release a NEW book, we offer it first to a small number of people as a test - drive. Because of your commitment here in downloading my book, I'd love for you to be a part of this group. You can join easily here → http://rapidslimdown.com/

"Shield your body to prevent diseases..."

Table of Content

Preface

"We can make a commitment to promote vegetables and fruits and whole grains on every part of every menu. We can make portion sizes smaller and emphasize quality over quantity. And we can help create a culture-imagine this-where our kids ask for healthy options instead of resisting them" - Michelle Obama.

"Being in control of your life and having realistic expectations about your day-to-day challenges are the keys to stress management, which is perhaps the most important ingredient to living a happy, healthy and rewarding life"- Marilu Henner.

Being in control of your life is what matters; this is undoubtedly what we should all adhere to. And it is not impossible to attain it. It is not a utopian concept. So, each one of us can do our part and make this world a better place for ourselves as well as for our children. After all, how many of us can actually see our children get obese and wait in queue to get a bariatric surgery done!!

As there is an old saying, "charity begins at home". What you do will be imbibed by your kids. So, get set for a healthy you where you can shed that odd looking flab around your waist and get ready to get a new lease of life. For this, you have to do a bit of homework as we all know that there are no shortcuts in life and there are no free lunches. So, even if you are fending for yourself, you can "free yourself" of those heavy lunches to emerge as a new you!!

Chapter 1

IT BEGINS HERE

Every time you bite into your favorite flavored cupcake, you experience heaven. But once you gulp it down, you wish you hadn't eaten it! This is a common phenomenon that occurs in almost all weight conscious people. Also, most of us believe that all the health conscious foods don't taste good. But this is gradually being proven wrong. With the advent of diets like the Bulletproof Diet, you can stay fit, and achieve great health, while enjoying sumptuous dessert, recipes, and menus that you can't get enough of! We will come to the recipe and lip smacking bulletproof meal plans later in the book. But it is important to understand the concept of bulletproof diet, if you really want to benefit from this and if you want to see yourself with the perfect vital statistics a couple of years from now! So, let's get going!

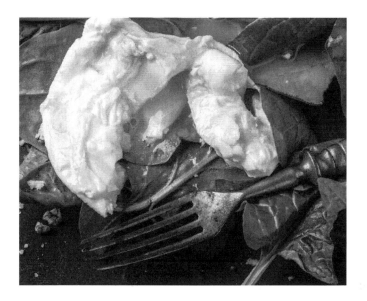

I. The First Step – Understanding the Basics

The mantra of success of the bulletproof diet is that you have to eat the right kind of foods that will ensure that you stay lean without losing muscle mass, and at the same time you should be oozing with energy.

Embarking upon this kind of diet does not necessarily mean that you will compromise on your immune system. While you are on the diet, you should be in great health too and not fall ill with cough, common cold, and other ailments. This implies that your resistance power should not be forsaken.

The underlying concept of the bulletproof diet is that the calories that you ought to take in daily, out of which 50% to at least 60% of the calories should be obtained from healthy fat, rest should be obtained from vegetables and protein.

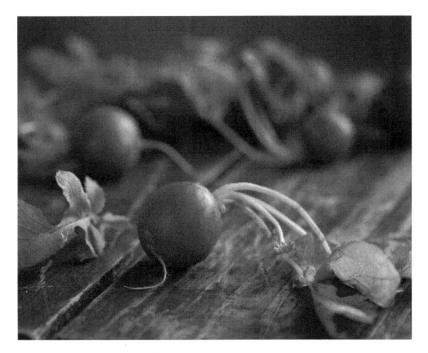

If you are surprised to read that the majority of the caloric intake should come from fat, you can relax because this time around, you can consider fat not as a fattening agent but as a component of the diet that will help you to lose weight. You can bank upon a particular variety of fat that essentially includes items such as avocados, coconut oil, butter, and of course, meat.

When adapting to the Bulletproof diet, you don't have to be extra cautious. No need to worry because you will be eating the right kind of food. Self restraint is important. You may feel the urge to indulge in food items that you are not supposed to have, comfort yourself and try to focus on the objective of the bulletproof diet. It is a pity that many individuals fail to derive the maximum benefits from this diet because they leave the diet regime midway because they lack perseverance.

To gain the maximum benefits of the diet, combine it with some exercise. Weight lifting can be one option. Alternatively, fast intervals are also helpful. And if at all you have doubt about the type of exercises that can help you to complement the diet, you can always seek expert advice.

Generally speaking, bulletproof diet will include all the major meals, namely, breakfast, lunch, and dinner. While you can take eggs and bacon, omelet, and vegetables for breakfast, you can take soup made of all your favorite vegetables added with some spice, butter, and nuts for taste for lunch. Remember, the bacon and eggs you take for breakfast should essentially be from pastured animals. For dinner, it would be a mix of carbs, proteins, and vegetables.

So, you can try out different combinations of all the components mentioned.

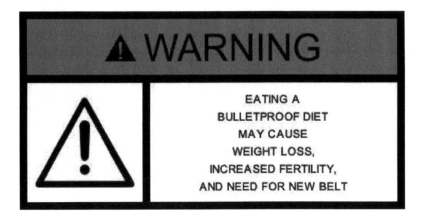

II.Intensify with Bulletproof Adaptation

What is a perfect healthy life? Although we know that there is nothing called a perfect life, this diet lets you get closer to it. Bulletproof diet is the stepping stone for a healthy life. As your Intelligent Quotient increases, you are able to deal with stress in a much better way, you don't become vulnerable to diseases, and you are able to perform all duties in a hassle-free manner. An ideal diet should be able to work wonders for your brain and body, while providing optimum nutrition.

What to expect from this diet?

The bulletproof diet will help you in a number of ways, namely,

- It will curb your cravings and constant hunger pangs

- Make your brain work in an optimum manner

- Provide immense physical and mental strength

- Enhance your determination to fight obesity

Remember, this diet is not just meant for the ones that are obese or overweight. If you have a hunch that your weight is getting out of control, you can start the diet right away and prevent further harmful fat from accumulating in your body.

This diet will help you to consume the right kind of food and most importantly the right quantity of food. The diet chart comprises of high content of fat, along with organic vegetables, and proteins in moderate amount. This diet should not only help you in weight loss, but should also offer sufficient energy. Expect this diet to positively impact your body and mind.

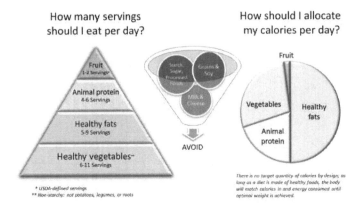

How many servings should I eat per day?

How should I allocate my calories per day?

* USDA-defined servings
** Non-starchy: not potatoes, legumes, or roots

There is no target quantity of calories by design; as long as a diet is made of healthy foods, the body will match calories in and energy consumed until optimal weight is achieved.

Balance micro and macronutrients

Starting the bulletproof diet plan does not mean that you will deprive your body of all the necessary nutrients. Vitamins and minerals are equally important. So, in order to get the best results, try your best to strike a balance between the macronutrients and the micronutrients that your body requires. Remember, it is not a wise move to weigh what you are eating when you start a new diet only in terms of calories. You have to listen to your body's needs. So, you must be wondering how you can lose weight by eating fat? You don't have to be scared. This is because you are eating the right kind of fat and not the type that will make you bloat up in an unhealthy manner.

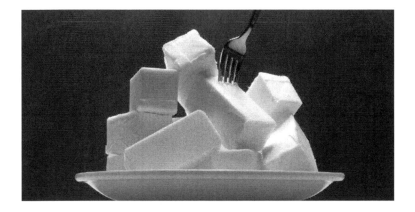

Fat is essential

One of the requirements of this diet is that you ought to eat meat of large animals that thrive on grass. Grass fed meat is natural and it is rich in nutrition. Opt for organ meat, if possible. It will help you to have healthy fat and meat. You cannot ignore fat completely. This is because, our body needs several vitamins like A, E.D. and these vitamins require fat to get dissolved and to be absorbed by the body.

Grains are to be avoided by all means, the classical examples being corn, millet, wheat, sorghum, barley, and oats. Such high carb food items tend to make you fat since they contain high levels of toxin, low nutrient content, and high sugar. The bulletproof diet will naturally remove all toxins from your body.

III. Seeing the Difference Firsthand!

Once you start the bulletproof diet regime, you will be surprised to witness the change in you. This holds true not just from the physical point of view but also mentally. As far as the physical effects are concerned, you become lean, you gain muscle mass (or at least do not lose it), you are super active, and most importantly, you are no longer among the category of people that have been labeled as belonging to high risk categories for diabetes, heart disease, cancer, and a number of other ailments.

A little bit of exercise (the right kind) will have a positive impact on your body while you are on this diet. It has been observed that there are many individuals that participate in marathons only to hurt themselves even more. This is because they do the exercise in a wrong manner that causes more harm than good. Exercise has a positive impact on muscles, sensitivity to insulin and other hormones in the body. It improves bone density, elevates mood, prevents mood swings, and enhances your overall well being.

One of the wrong ideas that most of us harbor within us is that exercise will help in burning fat. It may be mentioned here that hormones determine the body composition and not how much calories you are consuming. As such, you should exercise not to shed fat but to assist the hormones to manage calories effectively.

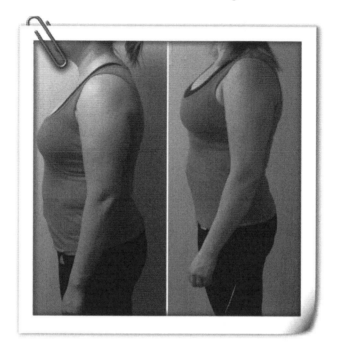

When you include bulletproof diet, gradually you notice positive changes in your body. But as mentioned above, the key points must be taken into account, which includes exercising to assist hormones to burn calories. You not only lose fat, but you also become sturdy and more energetic.

When you start a bulletproof exercise regime to complement the bulletproof diet, make sure, it is vivid, of shorter duration (brief), safe, and meaningful. In a nutshell, bulletproof diet affects your body in the following manner:

- Increases energy

- Improves sleep pattern

- Curbs appetite and harmful cravings

- Provides optimum balance of macro as well as micro nutrients

- Helps you to get accustomed to healthy way of eating

- Helps in burning calories the right way

Once you start, you will gradually get to see the benefits of this remarkable diet regime. Here are few more of these benefits that will make your efforts worthwhile.

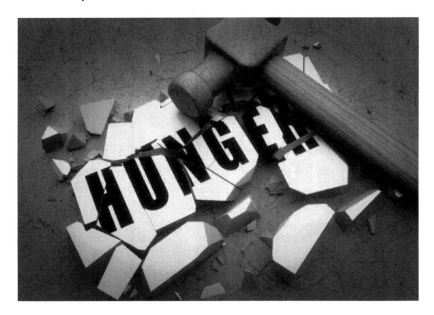

IV. The Perks You Can't Ignore

Bulletproof diet has changed the lives of many individuals. Aside from being one of the top avenues of weight loss, staying on this diet for a considerable period of time and abiding by the precepts and norms have proved to be beneficial for the entire body and mind. Given below are few changes that individuals undertaking the diet declared.

- Weight loss was observed in individuals that adhered well to the diet. This essentially means that daily the calorie intake should be 50% to 60% from fat, around 20% from protein, and the rest from vegetables. The ones that took the diet, recipes, and meal plans seriously were able to lose weight effectively.

- Staying on the bulletproof diet will also help you to reduce toxins from the body. This is because this diet is said to minimize mycotoxins.

- As far as weight reduction is concerned, this diet form reduces fat in the most "absurd" region of the body. Fat in the abdominal region is the hardest to remove. But in case of bulletproof diet, you will find that this area shows marked improvement first.

- There is gain in muscle mass and loss in fat

- There is overall improvement in the percentage of fat. This means that even if you find that there is increase in weight, it means that fat mass is reducing, muscle mass is improving. It means that the body is gradually developing proper fat composition, which is healthy.

- Staying on the diet also has impact on the biomarkers. Essential parameters like cholesterol, triglycerides, LDL, HDL, showed improvement.

- It will address issues of hunger pangs and food cravings. Binge eating is harmful and can increase your weight unnecessarily, which is not desirable.

- Needless to mention that if the biomarkers are also taken care of by the bulletproof diet, your chances of falling sick and getting cardiac disease, and lifestyle related diseases like hypertension, and other allied problems minimize to a great extent.

- People suffering from sleep disorders often need to rely on sleep medications. The bulletproof diet changes things for the better. It improves circadian rhythm, and helps you sleep better.

- Last but not the least, other weight loss diet regime will require you to stop all fatty foods and few of them also require you to skip meals. But thanks to the bulletproof diet, you can eat healthy fatty food, and you can also continue taking your favorite desserts.

This eBook offers a whole new range of recipes and meal plans that you can check out. Also, you can start your day with your favorite coffee. The only difference is that the bulletproof coffee will kick start your day and you can stay energetic and rejuvenated throughout the day to take on life anew!

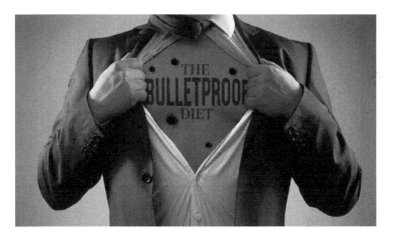

V. Watch Your Back for Pitfalls

Just as every coin has got two sides, when you are opting for the bulletproof diet, you must be prepared to accept the pitfalls too. This is because the rate of metabolism differs from one individual to another. So, if this diet is suitable for you, it may not be fit for someone else. It has been observed that this type of diet may not give you optimum results under the following circumstances-

- **Counting calories won't help this time around** - If you are too calorie conscious, the rules of this diet may seem absurd to you. Unlike the other forms of diet, where you have to pay heed to the number of calories you are consuming, this diet puts focus on eating right. Keep in mind that if you try to work out things in your own way, you will not reach anywhere. Abide by the norms of the bulletproof diet only. Stick to the foods that you are supposed to eat, even if that means eating a high fat diet.

- **Previous ailments and disorders** - This diet may not work for you if you have other health issues. Prior to starting the diet, it is important that you address those issues, and then try to reduce weight through this diet plan. It is essential for you to keep in mind that the rate of metabolism is not the same in case of every individual. If you have been suffering from any other ailment, you may not get the same results. So, it is of utmost importance that you check out with your doctor before you start the bulletproof diet. There are certain conditions that might hamper your chances of obtaining optimum results from this diet plan. These include hormonal imbalances, micronutrient deficiencies, chronic stress, and severe accumulation of toxins, anomalous circadian rhythms and so on.

- **Deviation from bulletproof diet** - This is of course quite obvious that if you do not follow the diet plan, meals, and recipes in an appropriate manner, you will not get the desired result.

- **Increased levels of cholesterol-** Few reports suggest that individuals that had taken to bulletproof coffee had elevated levels of cholesterol, which is again a precursor to heart ailment in many individuals.

VI. Are You the Right Candidate?

Whether you are the right candidate or not for this type of diet will be best decided by your GP. At no point of time should you start the bulletproof diet all by yourself. Disappointing as it may sound, this is the fact. Your GP knows about your body's dietary requirements much better than you do. This holds especially true if you are already suffering from few ailments like diabetes, hypertension, cardiac ailments, nerve disorders, and so on.

Also, you ought to consult your medical practitioner if you are breastfeeding/nursing/lactating, pregnant, and suffering from hormonal imbalance. This is because each one of our bodies behaves in a different manner to changes in diet and exercises. So, if you have achieved your target weight loss within the time expected, someone else may have taken a longer time to achieve the same target. So, it is relative and it is best to carry out certain tests prior to starting the bulletproof diet.

If you want to see how your metabolism and body composition has changed after you have started the diet, these tests can help you to mark the changes. This can be better understood with the help of an example. For instance, an individual that wanted to join the bandwagon of people adopting the bulletproof diet underwent various tests that included DXA scan, which measures body composition. Aside from this the individual underwent tests for kidney, liver, lipid panel, and bone density markers. After he completed the bulletproof diet for a certain period of time, he found that certain health markers or parameters had risen while few had reduced and returned to the normal levels. So, it is best if you carry out these tests prior to beginning the bulletproof diet regime.

Chapter 2

MOVING ON

Once you gather the basic knowledge on the Bulletproof diet, it is time for you to move on to the next phase. Changing your dietary habits and sticking to a healthy diet plan takes effort. Oftentimes, you may feel lost and hopeless. Having a guide at hands helps a great deal in times like these. Here, you will find all information you need to make your transition into the following stages of adapting to the Bulletproof lifestyle.

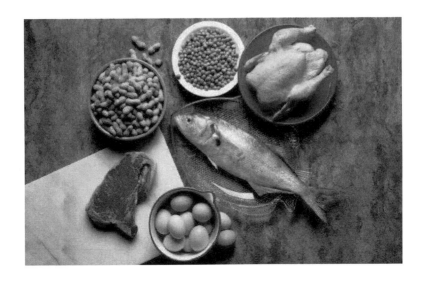

I. Guidelines You Must Follow

If you want to get the optimum result from the bulletproof diet, there are few guidelines that you must follow. Let us catch a glimpse of these guidelines in the following points.

- If you want longevity, you have to make an effort once a week. In this plan, you have to make sure that your protein intake does not exceed 25grams on that day. This is known as bulletproof protein fasting. It helps and is known as bulletproof protein fasting.

- There is another protocol called IF or Intermittent Fasting, which aids digestion and gives longevity. Once you have your bulletproof coffee, avoid eating anything before your lunchtime. This is called IF because you have something for breakfast, yet you fast until you feel hungry or till the lunchtime.

- It is best to eat only if you are feeling hungry. So, if it is lunchtime and you are still not feeling hungry, don't eat. Also avoid binge eating or snacking.

- If you are a woman, and you have to shed a lot of weight, you can add some protein with your bulletproof coffee. However, this practice will continue for the initial 60 days. And if at all you have to take protein, make sure it is from grass fed animals. Another alternative for pregnant women is the No Coffee Vanilla Latte recipe.

- Once you have completed 14 days (2 weeks) on the bulletproof diet, you enter the so called "maintenance mode". Now, you can add something else to your breakfast aside from just bulletproof coffee. You can opt for avocado, smoked salmon, or poached eggs.

- Bulletproof carbohydrates are also required and this means you have to add 30 grams of carbohydrate with vegetables. However the ideal time to take this combo is during the evening time. On the day you are fasting (IF), you can add 100 grams to 150 grams of carbohydrate to your diet. Remember, it is a proven fact that if you take less carbohydrate daily, you also lose weight fast. So, if you can limit your carbohydrate intake, it will complement your effort to lose weight when you are on the bulletproof diet regime.

There are foods that you have to avoid completely, foods that you can limit intake of, and then again foods that you can eat without having to think about weight loss and whether or not you are on the right track.

- The main mantra of success of this bulletproof diet is that you should stop eating once you have achieved satiety. Don't force-feed.

- You must not count the calories but take in the right kinds of food.

- Use spices to your food preparation. You can use thyme and rosemary powders.

- Make use of low temperatures if you have decided to cook and use water when you cook freely. Avoid using microwave or frying your foods.

- Consume organic vegetables and fruits as much as possible.

- Avoid homogenized food, pasteurized dairy products, and processed food items.

- Legumes are to be avoided by all means

- Do not use colorings, additives, preservatives, and flavorings to your food.

If you follow all the general guidelines, the bulletproof diet should yield the desired results.

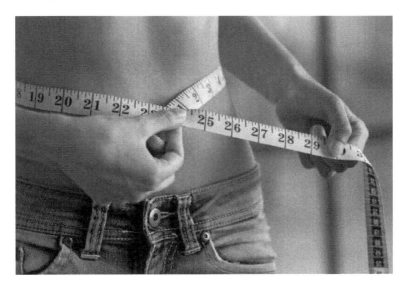

II. Bye-Bye Obesity!

If you have opted for the bulletproof diet, you surely want to look your best by losing the flab around your waist. Remember, losing weight also makes you look younger and fresh. You have a lot of energy at your disposal. All you have to do is follow the rules of the diet and your efforts are sure to bear fruit. Here we will take a look at the finer aspects of the diet so that you can shed weight effectively and say Bye-Bye Obesity! Pay heed to the following points-

•   Gluten is harmful, and known to cause inflammation. Also, flow of blood to the cerebral area is minimized when you consume too much of gluten. Most importantly, if it does not help you in losing weight, you should cut out gluten from your diet.

•   Consuming grass fed products is better. Also, it is best if you limit your intake of dairy protein (from cheese as well as milk).

•   Avoid taking starch just before you sit for your dinner. Sugar products should also be curtailed before dinner. This causes your blood sugar levels to fluctuate. As a result of which there are food and hunger cravings, which is not good when you are on the bulletproof diet. However, if you can take starch moderately during the dinnertime, it can improve your sleep greatly.

•   If you are into cooking, make sure you don't use olive oil or canola oil. Instead, coconut oil or butter from grass fed animals is a better choice.

•   Earlier, it was believed that egg yolk is not good for your health. But when you are on bulletproof diet, you can take

the yolk. This is because yolk aids in building myelin. This is the lining of the nerves. Aside from that, the good cholesterol known as HDL is found in the egg yolk. Besides, having yolk also improves hormones.

- High intensity coupled with low repetition exercises will give you a bulletproof body.

- Avoid using too much of MCT oil. This oil aids the Krebs cycle. This in turn produces ATP or Adenosine triphosphate cellular energy.

- If you consume fat at the beginning of the day, it helps you in doing away with stress. Also, it facilitates fat burning mode.

- If you incorporate collagen in your diet, it helps in improving the artery lining.

- Bulletproof coffee helps in weight loss. The coffee will "feed" the bacteria that will aid in weight loss.

Gaining weight is always easy. Unless you are disciplined about what you eat, especially if you are trying to lose weight, you will take a lot of time to reach your goal. Try out this unique bulletproof diet if you want to lose weight. So, make the most of the bulletproof diet. Why waste your time and energy on other diet regime when you have this tested and tried diet plan right in front of you? Most importantly, the ones that have undertaken the diet have appreciated the diet and its simplicity. So, get set for a new you and watch your personality grow. All will certainly love your new look.

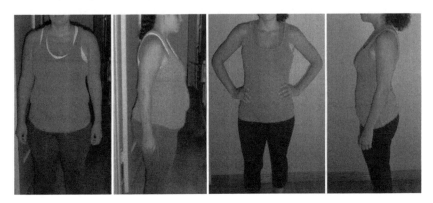

III. Bulletproof Rapid Loss Protocol Exists

You have already read about the basic concept and all the benefits and drawbacks of the bulletproof diet in the previous chapter. An important part of the bulletproof diet is the intermittent fasting and rapid fat loss protocol that helps not only to reduce the weight, but also to increase the levels of the mental energy.

What is the rapid fat loss protocol?

The Rapid Fat Loss Protocol is actually an important mode of losing weight that is being attempted by people following the bulletproof diet. This type of protocol is mainly being used by the people who wanted to lose their maximum amount of fat in the shortest span of time, without feeling weak. Bulletproof coffee improves the brain function, increases fat loss and keeps your stomach full for a long time to such an extent that you won't feel like eating till the afternoon. The Rapid Fat Loss Protocol combines modified cyclical bulletproof diet with mTOR stimulation, mitochondrial optimization, and ongoing toxin binding. The ultimate result is the massive rapid fat loss with fewer metabolic problems associated with the very low calorie diets.

Working of the Bulletproof Rapid Fat Loss Protocol

The Rapid Fat Loss Protocol is one of the main parts of the bulletproof diet, and it has been approved by professional dieticians as well. In the bulletproof diet, low carbohydrates are being consumed that causes the body to switch from the burning glucose to partly replacing it with the ketone bodies produced from the fats. The entire process is being carried over by the fatty-acid oxidation in the mitochondria level, which eventually leads to large amounts of acetyl-coA to be produced and generating the three important ketone bodies such as hydroxybutyrate, acetoacetate, and acetone. It is the job of all the ketone bodies to supply enough fuel for the rest of the body during the entire term of bulletproof diet.

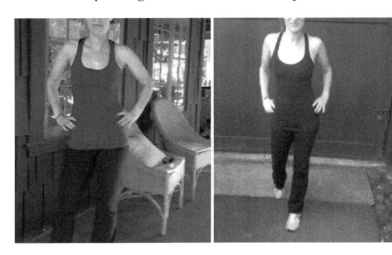

Step wise approach to the Rapid Fat Loss Protocol

The main goal of this protocol is to lose as much fat as possible as fast as possible using the very low calorie diets. Below are the primary steps that you need to follow.

Step 1: Before starting the protocol, it is better for you to eat a strict bulletproof diet for at least a week or two and store some extra nutrients in the body, which will help to reset your hormonal status. Another advantage is that after adapting to this diet you may not find it necessary to initiate your protocol anymore. You should go through a detailed blood test of your liver enzymes, vitamin D levels and blood lipids before starting the protocol.

Step 2: Drink the bulletproof coffee every morning. It is a mixture of brewed upgraded coffee beans along with grass-fed butter and brain octane oil that will eventually increase thermo genesis and ketone formation in the body. Try to drink as much as coffee as you can and not the other drinks. You can drink lots of water adding a pinch of salt or can eat butter with pink Himalayan salt on it. Do remember that you cannot eat any proteins or carbs.

Step 3: Do consume enough of vitamin supplements such as vitamin D3, magnesium, krill oil, vitamin k2, unbuffered vitamin C, branched chain amino acids, glutathione force, coconut charcoal, pink Himalayan salt.

Step 4: Re-feed yourself after at least 5 days of eating only fat food items and you will be in deep ketosis and burning only the fat. Re-feed helps as it resets the leptin level and prevent a large drop in the energy levels. Following this will eventually help you to sleep properly and will increase your mental strength and energy.

Step 5: Again re-examine all your blood tests to observe the difference it had, after following the protocol strictly. You will experience that HDL will be higher along with LDL, that is possible as the metabolic years of toxins stored in the body.

Try these steps and get ready to bank on the benefits right away!

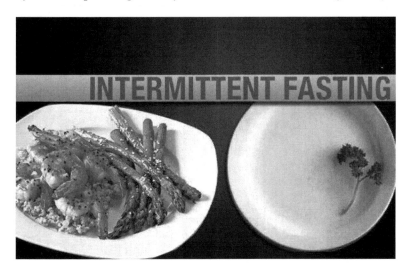

IV. Time to Adapt to Intermittent Fasting

The bulletproof diet is the best diet chart formulated not only to reduce weight, but also to increase mental energy. Intermittent fasting is one of the main methods of the bulletproof diet. The basic idea is to eat daily food in a shortened period and fast the rest of the time. This particular type of fasting differs much more than the regular fasting and will eventually bring a change in your entire lifestyle.

What is the intermittent fasting?

Most people believe Intermittent Fasting is a different diet form altogether, but it is wrong! Rather it is a pattern of taking meals in a day. People mainly try the intermittent fasting method in order to lose weight and also to keep muscle mass steady in the process of getting lean. It is one of the best strategies that help to take off the bad weight and maintain the good weight, which requires very little behavioral change. Intermittent fasting becomes effective when it comes to:

- Reducing blood glucose and insulin levels, and improving the state of the overall glucose metabolism in the body.

- Increasing fatty acid oxidation along with FFAs through increasing lipolysis hormones GH, glucagon and adrenalin.

- Keeping metabolism strong and healthy

- Addressing various health factors such as lowering inflammation and blood pressure, while reducing oxidative stress and increasing protection against nervous problems and diseases.

- Preserving muscle tissues

How does the intermittent fasting work?

In order to understand the working procedures of intermittent fasting, it is important to be aware of the differences between the fed state and the fasted state.

Fed state - During the digestion and absorption food items, the human body remains in the fed state. It is really difficult for the body to burn fat, as the insulin levels remain high.

Fasted state - After a specific time span, the body passes onto the stage of post-absorptive state that lasts from 8 to 12 hours after the last meal. Then the body enters into the fasted state. It is actually easy to burn fat in this fasted state as insulin levels remains very low. But you need to wait for 12 hours after the last meal to get into the fasted state. This is one of the key reasons behind many people fail to follow the intermittent fasting method.

Why the intermittent fasting does work better than the others?

Tripling down on mTOR: Mammalian Target of Rapamycin or mTOR is a major mechanism that increases protein synthesis in the body muscles.

Ketosis: ketosis is the fat burning mode that is good for the brain. The plain intermittent fasting helps you to enter the mode of ketosis and it will end if you eat carbs containing foods at the end of the fast.

You will love doing it: Intermittent fasting is appropriate for people who lead a normal life and work hard throughout the day. Intermittent fasting consists of bulletproof coffee and that is what makes it more enjoyable than the other fasting methods.

Metabolic hacking: Bulletproof coffee increases the body's metabolism up to 20%, which in turn will add further benefits to the body.

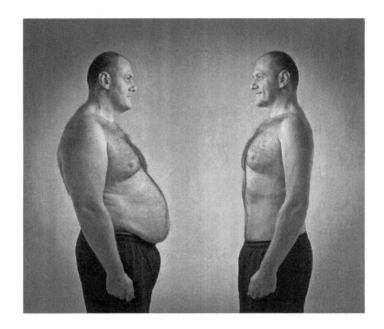

V. There are no ifs in IF!

As you start the bulletproof diet intermittent fasting, you will feel the change in yourself within few weeks. The fasting protocol not only changes you physically and makes you slim, but it will also change your level of energy, making you feel much more active. The fasting is easy to follow and maintain throughout a long period of time. On the whole, if you want to lose fat and improve health in a short span of time, intermittent fasting is the way to go! Here are some of the benefits that you can derive from practicing the intermittent fasting method:

✓ **Intermittent fasting makes your day much simpler**: This fasting offers additional simplicity to your life. When on fast, you don't need to worry about breakfast and other heavy meals. The fasting will allow you to eat only one meal. Therefore, there is lesser need to cool and plan meals. All these factors together make life much simpler and enjoyable.

✓ **Intermittent fasting helps you to live longer**: Long ago, scientists and researchers had already stated the fact that restricting calories is a way of lengthening the cycle of life. But there is no one who will wish to starve in order to live longer. By implementing intermittent fasting in your life, you will be hitting the right balance between eating and starving, which will offer a plethora of benefits.

✓ **Reduces the risk of cancer:** Although it is debatable, many researchers believe that intermittent fasting helps in reducing the probability of cancer. Studies reveal that fasting before the treatment may diminish the side effects of chemotherapy. Intermittent fasting not only reduces the risk of cancer, but it also prevents cardiovascular diseases.

✓ **Easier to follow**: Many times diet does not work out as we fail to stick into our respective diet chart for a long time. This is not a problem in the case of intermittent fasting as it is easy to implement and follow.

✓ **Positive effects**: While following the intermittent fasting, serum formed in the body had positive effects on the human epitome cells. It reduces triglycerides in men and increases HDL in women and also reduces the cell proliferation and increased heart resistance power. It may also function as a form of nutritional hormesis.

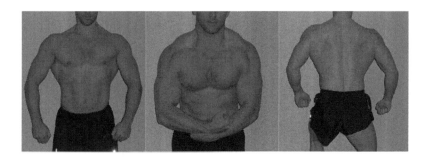

The effects of intermittent fasting on performance:

Intermittent fasting may have negative effects on the aerobic and anaerobic measures. In addition to that, the fasted athletes may face higher levels of fatigue during their training period but may not face a decrease in performance or strength.

Effects of intermittent fasting on the emotional status of mind:

People, who are strictly maintaining intermittent fasting schedule, may experience a decrease in emotional eating and a rapid increase in restrictive eating. It gets regularized after a certain period of time and simultaneously the body gets adjusted with the diet.

Effects of intermittent fasting on the body composition:

In the present world, calorie restriction through intermittent fasting might be as effective as the continuous restriction that is the most common dieting format. It is a fact that a decreased metabolic rate eventually slows down the weight-loss train and thus reduces the weight.

Chapter 3

LOSING WEIGHT – YOU'RE ALMOST THERE!

The Bulletproof Diet is all about maintaining the balance between the right amount of food and the right type of food. When you start practicing a bulletproof diet, remember that this diet is based entirely on the high amounts of healthy fats, moderate amounts of high quality protein and loads of vegetables. You should eat all these at the right time and in the right amount to reduce weight. Precisely, based on the scientific evidences and personal experimentation, the bulletproof diet is not merely a diet but a lifestyle.

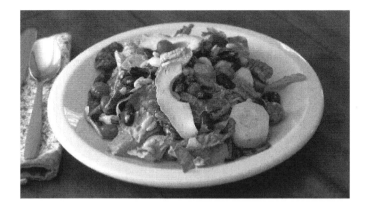

I. **Bulletproof Diet - a Necessity**

The bulletproof diet is necessary in the present world as it removes the anti nutrients or toxins from the food list, and endorses only healthy fats, vegetable and proteins. It may sound surprising to you, but following this particular diet chart, you can actually lose a pound a day in 2 weeks and that too without staying hungry. Apart from that, following the diet will allow your skin to glow, hair to strengthen and energy levels to increase.

You can also build up a healthy and toned body in your 40s, which is a remarkable achievement at this age. This is possible because as you can shed off the excess pounds from your body and concentrate on eating healthy fats such as avocados, eggs, olive oil, nuts, nut butter and fatty fish.

Many people do heavy workouts along with the diet in order to reduce weight fast. But the bulletproof diet is effective even on people who don't like exercising. However, combining exercises with the diet will show the results significantly faster. The primary bulletproof exercises include seated row, chest press, pull down, overhead press and leg press.

When adapting to the bulletproof lifestyle, you can cut down on the unnecessary supplements that do more harm than good. However, experts recommend few dietary supplements including:

- Vitamin D

- Magnesium

- Vitamin K2

- Vitamin C

- Iodine

- Krill Oil (EPA/DHA)

- Vitamin A

This diet can be especially beneficial for pregnant women as it low in sugar and high in healthy fats, essential for the developing fetus. The sugar levels affect hormone levels and cause a threat to fertility.

I'm not Dieting I'm changing my Lifestyle ♡

II. A Friend for Life?

Undoubtedly, bulletproof diet is one of the healthiest and the most nutritious diet. Oftentimes, we begin following a diet with the desire to lose weight, and when we achieve our goal, we fall off the wagon and start eating unhealthy again. If you wish to maintain your perfectly fit body, breaking the dietary rules will not help. In such cases, the body clock revolts back, and takes you back to where you had started.

Bulletproof diet has garnered popularity not just because it offers miraculous weight loss. People swear by this diet because it changes their lifestyle for the better. Here are some of the facts that would make you want to make this diet your friend for a lifetime:

- You can reduce weight and create your own path of healthy living

- You can lose weight with zero hunger and zero cravings for food

- You will be in control of both your mind and body

- You can enjoy nuts, dark chocolate, avocado and butter, and have them fight off diseases!

- You will have newfound energy, motivation and drive for life

If you wish to reach your desired weight, and remain slim and trim for life, start the bulletproof diet and get ready to see the difference.

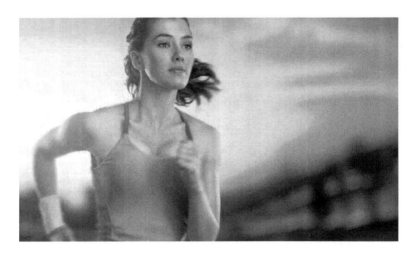

III. How to Shed 1 Pound per Day?

Did you know that the bulletproof diet allows you to lose 1 pound every day? It may sound almost impossible, and even utopian! But it does not change this fact that many people have reported. Unlike the regular diets, bulletproof diet removes anti nutrients or toxins from the food list and makes you eat only healthy fats, vegetable and proteins. When combined with intermittent fasting, this diet can be truly rewarding. The initial process of bulletproof fasting is to consume a cup of bulletproof coffee in the morning.

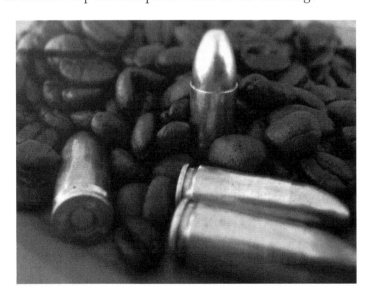

Main ingredients of the bulletproof coffee:

- Grass fed butter and MCT oil: Supplies the stable current of energy in the body that will keep you fresh throughout the day.

- Upgraded coffee beans: These coffee beans are ultra low toxin which optimizes the brain function and causes fat loss due to the presence of high octane caffeine.

- MCT oil: Increases the ketone production and enhances the metabolic rate by up to 12%.

- XCT oil: This is an additional ingredient, which will promote the ketogenesis and provide the person with a mental kick.

Bulletproof coffee fills up the stomach to such an extent that you won't feel like eating till the afternoon. Thus it helps to restrict hunger and reducing weight. But you shed single pound in day accurately if you strictly follow the green side of the bulletproof diet along with the fasting protocol. Therefore the secret of shedding a pound in a day is not any treasure hunt but the secret is hidden in your daily lifestyle. You can achieve this by sticking to your diet, following the fasting rules, and doing the right exercises.

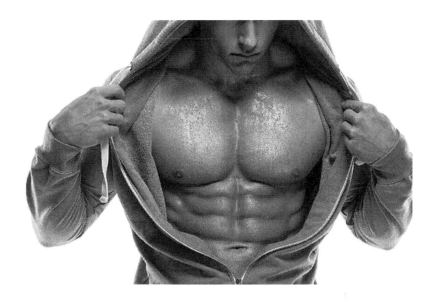

IV. Make Your Body Bulletproof!

You may spend hours in the gym, working out rigorously to remain strong and sturdy. But all of these efforts will go in vein if you fail to eat healthy. Instead of focusing only on exercising, make sure you create a perfect combination of dieting and exercising. When you are able to blend these two components, you would be rewarded with a bulletproof body that is not only attractive, but is also shielded against diseases. Find out how you can shape the bulletproof way:

- **Eat according to the bulletproof diet:** Following the strict bulletproof diet will help you to maintain the muscles mass, reduce fat, avoid diseases and delay aging. The bulletproof diet is about what to eat and how to eat which eventually determines the body composition.

- **Avoid toxins:** This is one of the main reasons that make bulletproof diet stand out from the other diets. Xenoestrogens, mycotoxins and other substances can act as "obesigens" that will help to produce fat.

- **Get proper sleep:** Proper sleep is the main aspect of the maintaining a bulletproof body. Without sleep, body won't repair muscle tissue, burn fat or recover for the following day. If you do regular exercises, you require more sleep. Improper sleep causes cortisol imbalance and long term endocrine damage.

- **Follow the exercise guide:** Although exercise is not the only way to achieve a bulletproof body, it can improve bone density, mood, and blood lipids, while increasing insulin sensitivity. Body composition is determined by the hormones and not by the amount of calories. Exercise is not the method to burn calories. Rather it influences the hormones effectively. Points to be remembered in case of exercise:

a. Don't over-exercise, as more exercise does not always lead to more benefits.

b. Do not perform more than one exercise session per week if you fail to give optimum time for sleep.

c. Exercise sessions should not be more than 20 minutes in very high intensity.

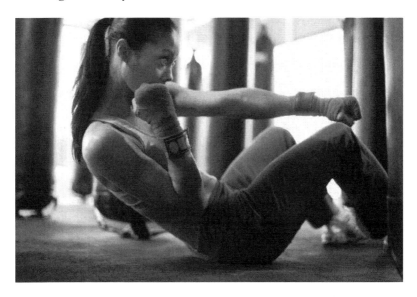

V. Get. Set. Go!

The bulletproof diet is not a particular diet chart but the lifestyle, which should be practiced sincerely. It will take some for the results to be noticeable, as your body requires time to become accustomed to the new metabolism cycle. Frankly speaking, you will feel the effects within 2 to 4 weeks after starting the diet. The main aim of the bulletproof diet is creating high levels of energy in the body, and reducing weight effectively. In the process, you need avoid carbohydrates and eat the right kind of fats and calories. Here is the stepwise approach to start on the bulletproof diet:

- Eliminate sugar

- Opt for healthy fats such as grass-fed butter, ghee, MCT and coconut oil.

- Remove all the synthetic additives, colorings and flavorings from your food list.

- Eat major amount of pastured and grass-fed meat such as beef, lamb and bison

- Don't forget items such as fish, eggs and shellfish.

- Eliminate gluten

- Avoid legumes like peanuts, beans and lentils (if you wish to take beans, make sure you soak them and sprout them before cooking)

- Eliminate grains, grain derived oils, and vegetable oils from the food list

- Try to switch to organic fruits and vegetables to improve immunity

- Remove all the processed, normalized and pasteurizes dairy from your diet

- Avoid fried products and cooking in microwave

- Eat lots of poultry eggs along with the pork, chicken, turkeys and ducks

- Add spices and herbs to make food tastier

- Learn to limit your fruit intake to 1-2 servings each day. Concentrate on low fructose containing fruits such as berries and lemons instead of watermelon and apples.

In order to be prepared for the bulletproof diet, do remember some of the key points while following the diet:

- Never count the calories in order to lose weight. Just enjoy your food

- Curb your desires to munch on junk food

- High healthy fat intake is optimal, and the general ranges of the fat are 50-80 percent fat, 5-30 percent carbohydrate and 10-30 percent protein.

- Supplement your food with fish oil or krill oil if you do not consume salmon on a weekly basis

The experts have observed it and professionals that the stepwise approach towards the state of bulletproof diet strengthens and improves brain functions. The more you cling on to this diet, the more you will become immune to all the diseases. Adapt to the bulletproof lifestyle, follow the rules, maintain the dos and don'ts of the diet, and start enjoying a healthy happy life!

Chapter 4

MEASURES TO TAKE

Initially in the beginning of the bulletproof diet, you may become confused regarding your types of food intake, as the concept is entirely new to you. This list of food items jotted down for you will eventually help you to be aware of which kinds of food you should consume and which are the foods you should avoid partially and completely. Most people are busy in their personal and professional life, and they do not have time to exhaust their mind on the diet chart on a regular basis. It's also very confusing to remember all the dos and don'ts of the diet chart. Therefore this list of foods of the bulletproof diet is being listed in order to help you to sort the foods you can eat without any anxiety of weight put on and the ones that you should avoid to remain healthy and fit throughout your life.

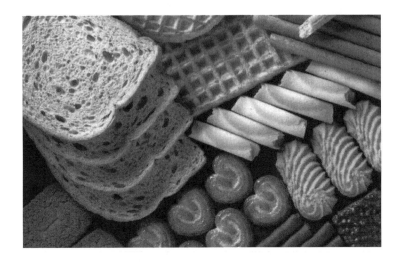

I. Foods You Should Fight Shy Of:

The bulletproof diet is the foundation of the bulletproof body and bulletproof mind. The bulletproof diet contains food items that target 50%-60% of calories from the good fats, 20% from protein and the rest from the different kinds of vegetables. Just eat according to the food chart of the diet mentioned and lose your weight effortlessly and gain muscle with the right exercises. Mainly formed based on the findings of biochemistry and human performance, the bulletproof diet is absolutely scientific, and it overcomes different problems that arise due to unhealthy food intake and lifestyle.

Given below is the list of protein foods items that you should avoid in a bulletproof diet:

- Soya protein

- Wheat protein

- Beans

- Cheese

- Other pasteurized or cooked dairy except butter

Here is the list of oil and fats, which you should avoid:

- Margarine

- Other artificial trans fats

- Oils made from GMO grains

- Corn oil

- Soy Oil

- Canola Oil

- Unstable polyunsaturated oils like walnut, flax and peanut oil

- Commercial lard

Among all the vegetables these are the specific ones, from which you should stay away always. They are:

- Potatoes

- Mushrooms

- Canned vegetables

- Vegetables with wilting or brown spots

Generally fruits are a part of the healthy diet, but in the case of bulletproof diet you should stay away from the canned fruits. Those contain preservatives and artificial sugar that causes to increase the weight and also lowers your energy level.

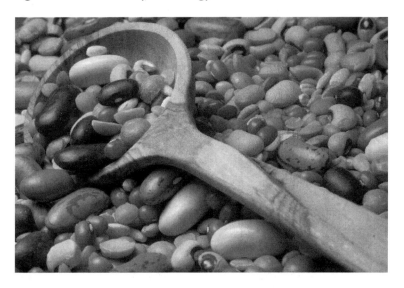

Nuts and legumes though are highly nutritious but some of them are absolutely restricted in the bulletproof diet such as:

- Non- fermented soy

- Soy Nuts

- Corn Nuts

- Roasted nuts

- Roasted legumes

Below listed are the grains that are to be avoided:

- Any kind of non organic refined or whole grains except rice

- GMO grain

The dairy products, which are to be avoided, are:

- Any dairy products from factory farms

- Any dairy products from farms using rBGH

- Powdered milk

- Condensed milk

- Ice cream

Spices and different types of flavorings are being used in many of the food products. Among all of which, some of them are being restricted:

- Commercial salad dressings

- Yeast

- Spice extracts

- Spices

- Flavoring

- Dyes

- MSG

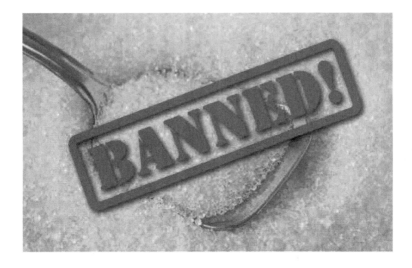

Generally, sweets and sweeteners are being advised against. The diet is very low in sugar and they are good in fighting inflammation, gut imbalances, candida issues or belly fat. The sweeteners that you should avoid are:

- Aspartame

- Sucralose

- Acelsulfame

- Agave syrup

- High fructose corn syrup

- Fruit juice concentrate

There are various methods of cooking food. Some of you may prefer deep fried whereas some prefer shallow fry. Many of you may think that microwave food is safe it requires little to no oil. The list of food items, which are to be avoided, had been listed but often in many diet charts, one point is generally ignored, that is the mode of cooking. In case of bulletproof diet, the method of cooking is also being specified in order to make it easier for you:

• Burnt

• Blackened

• Charred

• Deep Fried

• Microwaved

People often drink different kinds of soft drinks or sports drinks, being unaware of the fact that it is damaging the health. Of course, all the beverages can be taken sometimes but not regularly. Given below are the lists of beverages that are to be avoided completely in the bulletproof diet:

• Packaged juice

• Diet drinks

• Soda

• Sweetened drinks

• Aspartame drinks

• Sports drinks

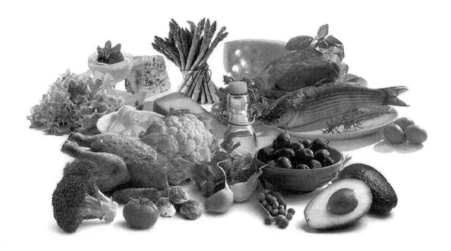

II.....And Foods You Can Devour!

The bulletproof diet actually teaches you to choose foods that provide the most energy and the most vitamins, yet contain the least amount of performance robbing, inflammation causing, anti nutrients and toxins.

Given below is the list of proteins that can be consumed regularly under a bulletproof diet:

- Grass-fed beef

- Grass-fed lamb

- Pastured Eggs

- Protein powders

- Hydrolyzed collagen

- Colostrum's Beef Plasma/Serum

- Pastured gelatin

- Organ meats from grass-fed animals such as liver (beef, lamb, goat, fish), kidneys, heart, tongue, bone marrow, joints (soup bones)

- Bulletproof collagen protein

- Whey protein concentrate

- Low mercury fish such as Anchovies, Haddock, Patrale, sole, sardines, sockeye salmon, summer flounder, Tilapia, Trout

The bulletproof diet advises to stop looking at fat as a fattening agent. And instead it embraces fat for the nourishment of the body. You will have much less stability in your hormones if there is lower intake of saturated fats. Some of the oils and fats, which you can consume, are:

- Grass-fed butter

- Bulletproof Brain Octane

- Grass-fed Ghee

- Pastured egg yolks (if you are not allergic to eggs)

- Krill Oil

- Virgin coconut oil

- Sunflower lecithin

- Grass-fed meat fat (bone marrow, tallow, lard, etc. but not poultry fat)

- Fish oils

- Coconut oil

- Bulletproof medium-chain triglyceride MCT oil

- Non-GMO soy lecithin

- Extra-virgin olive oil

- Bulletproof chocolate

- Chocolate butter

- Cocoa butter

- Avocado oil

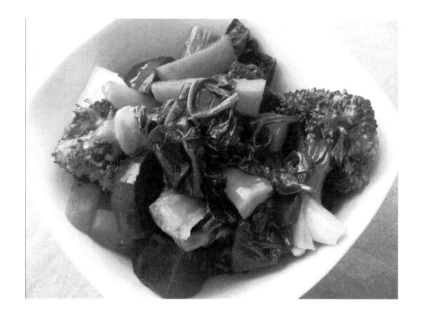

Vegetables are the important portions of the diet charts. Here is the list of vegetables approved by the bulletproof diet that you can consume without any fear of increasing weight.

- Avocados

- Cilantro

- Olives

- Parsley

- Bok Choy

- Brussels Sprouts

- Collards

- Cooked spinach

- Kale

- Asparagus

- Broccoli

- Cabbages

- Cauliflower

- Carrots

- Celery

- Cucumber

- Dark Lettuces

- Fennel

- Radish

- Artichokes

- Green beans

- Summer Squashes

- Zucchini

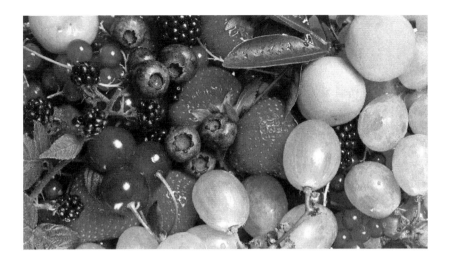

Many people do have fruits as a part of their breakfast, but they are unaware of the fact that it contains high amount of fructose that will not provide any long lasting energy boost. Rather they will cause more cravings for food and become the key reason behind increasing weight. Limit fruit consumption in order to avoid triglycerides. The bulletproof diet provides you with some of the low sugar fruits such as:

- Blackberry

- Cranberry

- Grapefruit

- Lemon

- Lime

- Passion Fruit

- Raspberry

- Strawberry

As far as nuts and legumes, here is the list given below in the case of bulletproof diet:

- Coconut Raw only

- Almonds

- Brazil nuts

- Cashews

- Hazelnuts

- Macadamia nuts

- Pecans

- Pine nuts

- Pistachios

- Walnuts

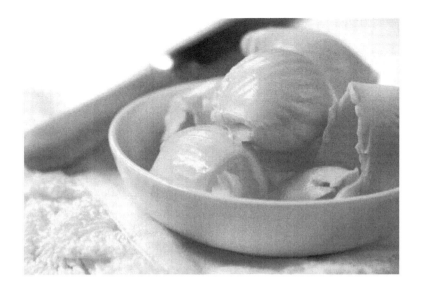

Dairy products are the important part of any diet chart. The bulletproof diet is different as they concentrate not only on the diet but also on the lifestyle of people. They suggest eating dairy products of grass-fed animals rather than grain-fed animals. The various dairy products that you can intake on a daily basis are as follows:

• Organic grass-fed butter

• Organic grass-fed ghee (clarified butter)

• Non-organic grass-fed butter

• Colostrum

• Non-organic grass-fed ghee

- Grass-fed full-fat raw organic milk (not pasteurized and only if tolerated)

- Grass-fed full-fat raw organic cream (not pasteurized and only if tolerated)

- Grass-fed full-fat raw organic yogurt (not pasteurized and only if tolerated)

The list of spices and flavorings that you can intake are being listed below:

- Apple cider vinegar

- Bulletproof Vanilla ax vanilla powder

- Sea salt

- Ginger

- Cilantro

- Parsley

- Oregano

- Turmeric

- Rosemary

- Lavender

- Thyme

- Cinnamon

- Bulletproof chocolate powder

- All-spice

- Cloves

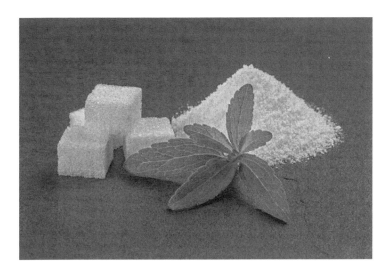

The bulletproof diet advises you not to consume sugar or starch before dinner as it increases your cravings for food. You can intake them in moderate amounts after food, some of them are listed below:

1) Xylitol (made from North American hardwood)

2) Erythritol

3) Stevia

4) Maltitol

5) Other sugar alcohols

6) Dextrose

There are various modes of cooking but do remember the fact that animal proteins are best eaten raw or rare, and grass-fed animals are less likely to contain parasites, pathogens, and toxins than those from grain-fed animals. Also it is being advised that cruciferous vegetables should be eaten cooked not raw. Some of the best ways of cooking are:

- Raw / Not cooked

- Lightly heated

- Steamed al dente

- Baked at 350oF or below

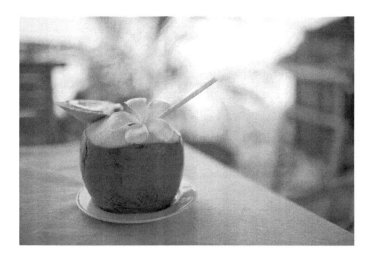

Beverages form an important part of our daily life. In the bulletproof diet chart, it occupies a vital position. Here are some of them, which are listed for you to clear your confusion of food intake:

- Coffee made from bulletproof upgraded coffee beans

- High quality green tea

- Diluted coconut milk (without carrageenan, preferably without guar gum, BPA free), do note that light coconut milk is just coconut milk plus water),

- Water with lime/lemon

- Mineral water in glass

- Fresh coconut water

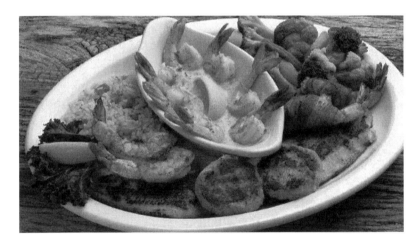

III. Then there Are Those to Take Moderately

Here is the list of some of the food items that you can consume once in a while or in a moderate manner but not on a regular basis. In other words these are the food items that are to be limited with the bulletproof diet. It is a fact that a person throughout the life cannot follow a strict diet chart. At times, you may have cravings for some other food items. The bulletproof diet gives you the liberty of eating some of these food items, but make sure you consume these items moderately.

There are some of the protein sources that can be consumed moderately but not on daily basis such as:

- Factory farmed eggs
- Pastured chicken, turkey, pork
- Pastured duck and goose
- Wild caught seafood
- Heated whey
- Hemp protein

Given below is the list of vegetables that you can include sometimes in your diet chart.

- Artichokes

- Green beans

- Carrots

- Cabbage

- Butternut and winter squash

- Leeks

- Green onion

- Parsley

- Peas

- Raw kale and spinach

- Raw collards

The lists of dairy products you eat sometimes are being listed below:

- Non-organic grass-fed full fat raw milk or yogurt

- Grain-fed ghee and butter

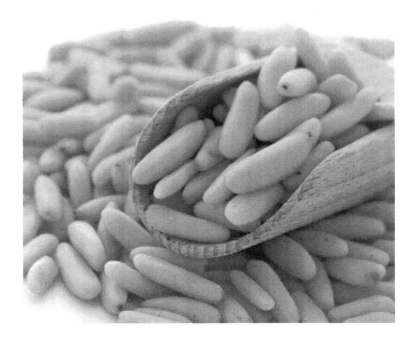

The list of nuts and legumes that are been included in the bulletproof diet on a moderate basis are given below:

- Pistachios

- Pine nuts

- Sprouted legumes

- Brazil nuts

- Dried peas

- Garbanzo beans

- Hummus

Spices and flavorings that are being marked as moderately used:

- Onion

- Table salt

- Mustard seed

- Garlic

- Paprika

- Nutmeg

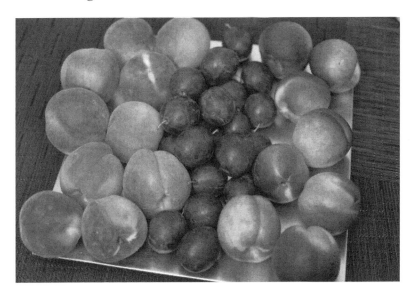

The Fruits included in the list are:

- Apple

- Apricot

- Cherries

- Kiwi

- Orange

- Peach

- Pears

- Plums

- Lychee

- Honeydew

- Grapes

- Papaya

If you do have a sweet tooth, then you can try some of these sweeteners moderately in a bulletproof diet:

- Maple syrup

- Coconut sugar

- White sugar

- Brown sugar

- Agave

- Cooked honey

Given below is the list of starch food items that can be used on an occasional basis:

- Black rice

- Wild rice

- Fresh or frozen organic corn on the cob

- Potatoes (white, purple new)

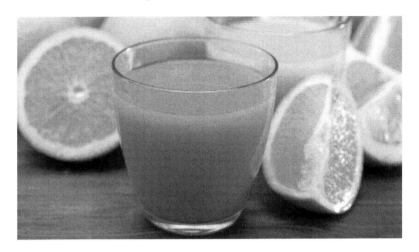

List of moderately taken beverages are:

- Kombucha

- Raw milk

- Bottled ice tea without sugar

- Coconut water

- Bottled nut milks

- Freshly squeezed fruit juice

The bulletproof diet mentions the detailing of the cooking method, so that it is easier for you to understand how to eat the above mentioned food items. These are some of the cooking methods, which you should use on a moderate basis such as:

- Sous vide

- Crock pot

- Boiled

- Barbequed

REPEAT AFTER ME:
"I CAN DO THIS"

IV. Staying Inspired, Staying Motivated!

It goes without saying that the bulletproof diet helps you achieve optimum health. However, in order to make the most of this diet, you would have to be determined to stick to it. The results will not be visible overnight. Getting frustrated and leaving the diet midway will not do you any good. That is why it is important for you to stay inspired and motivated. Here are some tips that you may find useful:

Get support from others: One of the best possible ways to stay motivated is to gather support from the ones who are already following the bulletproof diet plans. You can talk to them, understand how they are following the diet, what are their feelings and so on.

Learn about the scientific researches: The bulletproof diet is the result of years of research around human performance, cognitive function, fertility and anti-aging. It maintains healthy body without counting calories or starving.

Concentrate on the benefits rather than the drawbacks: The bulletproof diet has many benefits for which it is being named as one of the best diets. Great for meal planning and grocery shopping, the bulletproof diet explains everything right from the beginning.

Know about the health benefits: By implementing the bulletproof diet, you can reduce the risks of acne, brain fog, certain cancers, cardiovascular disease, diabetes, food cravings, gout, Hashimoto's disease, high triglycerides, inflammation, insulin sensitivity, migraine headaches, overweight/obesity and seasonal allergies.

Stick on to the bulletproof exercise: The bulletproof exercise is equally important to follow along with the bulletproof diet chart. It offers a number of advantages including weight loss, muscle build up, and toned muscles. Bulletproof exercise improves bone density, mood, blood lipids, and increases insulin sensitivity. It also helps to decrease inflammation and improves sleep.

Chapter 5

CAN YOU LET
THE BULLET IN?

Thinking of adapting to the bulletproof lifestyle? So far, you have learnt what this diet is all about, what sort of food items you should and shouldn't consume, and what kind of exercises you should include in your daily life. But there are few more important questions that may lurk in the corners of your mind. Some of these important aspects have been discussed below.

I. Is it safe for kids?

The bulletproof diet has been designed with proper scientific findings. Thorough research has been done to find out whether the diet is appropriate for all. However, when the question arrives on kids, it is always better to be in the safe side. It is better to consult a physician before introducing this diet to the kids. The metabolism powers of kids are different from that of an adult. Adding to that, they are also in a state of growth, which may require various types of nutrition. That is why it is crucial for kids to receive proper nutrition. In certain cases of childhood obesity, the bulletproof diet has shown significant benefits. However, the results may not be same for every kid. After a thorough checkup, your kid's physician will be able to tell you whether the bulletproof diet will be appropriate.

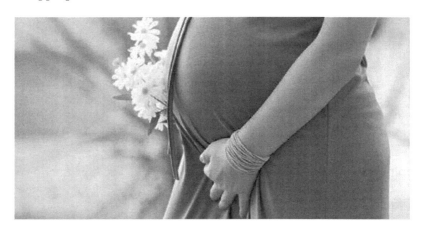

II.   What about Pregnant Women?

The bulletproof diet is related to primal, caveman or pale diets. The bulletproof diet is a balanced diet that consists of suitable amount of protein, healthy fats, and organic vegetables. The combination is a treasure trove of health for all individuals. But does it apply for pregnant women? Before beginning the bulletproof diet, pregnant women must consider the metabolic changes that their body will go through during the different stages of the pregnancy. The mother should consider the nutritional needs of the baby too. Before embarking on your bulletproof journey during pregnancy, make sure you consult your doctor about the complications that may arise due to the sudden change in the dietary routine.

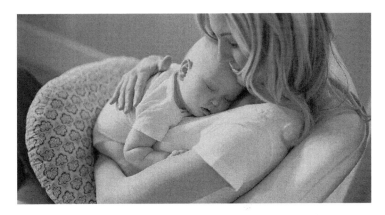

III. Appropriate for Nursing Mothers?

Are you eager to lose the extra weight you gained during pregnancy? If you are a fitness enthusiast, being overweight can seem like a torture! But starting a new diet right after childbirth may come with unwanted complications. Being a nursing mother, you have added responsibilities towards your child's nutritional needs. The first few months are crucial for a baby's growth, and breast milk is where the child derives nutrition. Starting a high fat, low carb diet may tamper with the nutritional value of the milk. You may even notice a reduced level in the production of milk. Because of all the possible complications, many experts advise nursing mothers to start dieting at least a few months after childbirth. However, if you are keen on starting the diet soon enough, make sure you consult your doctor to know if you can.

Chapter 6

RECIPES & MEAL PLANS TO MAKE IT EASIER

A dapting the regimen of Bulletproof Diet could be quite challenging. Several questions about selection of food could creep into your mind and you could be a victim of indecision. Therefore, in order to make things simple for you, I have prepared a ready to use meal plan for a fortnight so that you can make a head start instantly. Once the pace is set, you will find your own comfort level with the Bulletproof regimen and find enough encouragement to take it forward.

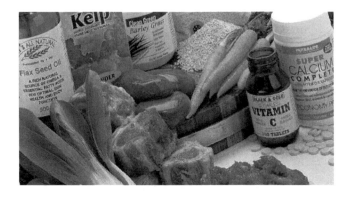

I. **Bulletproof Meal Plans**

When you make your own meal plan bear in mind the following guidelines:

- Abstain from consuming sugar in any form. Shun sports drinks and fruit juices that contain honey, agave and HFCS. Substitute sugar with healthy fats like butter (grass fed), ghee, olive oil or any other unheated oil and organic coconut oil. Healthy fats that are specially optimized can also be used.

- Switch over to grass fed and pastured meat - beef, bison and lamb. You can add seafood that is wild caught to this list.

- Stop using any kind of additives, flavorings and colorings that are synthetic in nature. Consuming any form of gluten is strictly prohibited too.

- Pasteurized, homogenized or processed dairy should be totally avoided.

- Say no to legumes like lentils, beans and peanuts.

- Focus on organic vegetables and foods.

- Limit the intake of fruits so as not to take more than two servings a day.

- Pay attention to gentle cooking at low temperatures and add spices to it.

So, here we go with the 14 Day Meal Plan that will initiate you into the world of Bulletproof diet.

Day 1

Breakfast: Bulletproof Pumpkin Spice Un-Latte

Lunch: Avocado and Salmon "Not Sushi"

Snacks: "Oh My Word" Bulletproof Chili

Beverages: Bullet Proof Manhattan Cocktail

Dinner: Chocolate Drizzled Pear Salad (with Lemon Rosemary Vinaigrette)

Desserts: Bulletproof Tiramisu

Day 2

Breakfast: Bulletproof Coffee

Lunch: Poached Eggs with Sautéed Greens

Dinner: Cauliflower-Bacon Mash

Day 3

Breakfast: Bulletproof Hot Chocolate Recipe

Lunch: Taco Salad

Snacks: Bulletproof Coconut Smoothies

Beverages: Bulletproof Coffee Knockoff

Dinner: Bulletproof Roast with Brussels Sprouts

Desserts: Berry Bowl

Day 4

Breakfast: Coffee Shake

Lunch: Bulletproof Satisfying Salad Dressing

Dinner: Roasted Lamb Rack with Cauliflower, Celery, and Fennel

Day 5

Breakfast: Bulletproof Luscious Latte

Lunch: Bulletproof Honey Mustard Vinaigrette

Snacks: Dark Chocolate Mud Cake

Beverages: Bulletproof green tea

Dinner: Pulled Pork Shoulder with Brussels Sprouts

Desserts: Chocolate Truffle Pudding

Day 6

Breakfast: Bulletproof Hot Chaga Chocolate

Lunch: Bulletproof Creamy Basil Vinaigrette

Dinner: Baked Fish with Steamed Butternut Squash

Day 7

Breakfast: Bulletproof eggs Benedict with bacon and Hollandaise sauce

Lunch: Bulletproof Ranch Dressing

Snacks: Bulletproof Coffee Pods

Beverages: Bulletproof Matcha Tea Smoothie

Dinner: Guacamole (Bulletproof)

Desserts: Coconut Ice Cream

Day 8

Breakfast: Bulletproof Maple Mocha

Lunch: Bulletproof Bone Broth Recipe

Dinner: Sweet Crockpot Pulled Pork

Day 9

Breakfast: Good Morning Granola with Orange-Infused Yogurt

Lunch: Bulletproof Shepherd's Pie

Snacks: Bulletproof Low Carb Fudgy Brownies

Beverages: Bulletproof Hot Cocoa

Dinner: Giant Stuffed Mushrooms

Desserts: Bulletproof Coffee Jelly Dessert

Day 10

Breakfast: Bulletproof Chai

Lunch: Penne all' Arrabbiata

Dinner: Primal Pot Roast

Day 11

Breakfast: Bulletproof Coffee Drops

Lunch: Penne alla Puttanesca

Snacks: Bulletproof Coffee Strawberry Cream Pops

Beverages: Bulletproof Latte Recipe

Dinner: Beef Burgundy

Desserts: Bulletproof MoJoe JingLato

Day 12

Breakfast: Bulletproof Pumpkin Frappuccino

Lunch: Chinese Lettuce Wrap

Dinner: Garlic Coconut Shrimp

Day 13

Breakfast: Blueberry Espresso Brownies

Lunch: Lettuce Wrap Grass Fed Burger

Dinner: Cashew Cheesecake Pie (Raw Vegan)

Day 14

Breakfast: Lemon Poppy Seed Muffins

Lunch: Chicken Pot Pie - The Sequel

Dinner: Bulletproof Fat Bombs

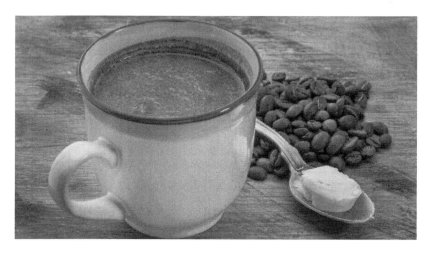

II. A Special Take on Bulletproof Coffee

Bulletproof Coffee is a coffee with a difference. Being different from all other types of coffee, it not only stands out from the rest but sets new standards of healthy diet that is based on the philosophy of consuming more healthy fats that would contribute to 50 -60% of calories that you need. So, what is so special about it? A cup of Bulletproof Coffee is all that you need to start your day with a bang. No more elaborate breakfast arrangements, just a few sips of Bulletproof Coffee and have your batteries recharged for the day.

It is not easy to get coffee without toxins. The manufacturing process contributes to the toxins that we find in coffee beans. Bulletproof Coffee beans are free from mycotoxins that cause anxious feelings and make you feel jittery. Therefore upgraded Bulletproof Coffee can give superb effects to your mental state that keeps you energized, lean and focused.

When you take Bulletproof Coffee you can be sure that you will get rid of your cravings for food. After all, it is this evil craving for food that tend sabotage your best intentions of following a healthy diet regime. It will give you a wholesome feeling, boost your energy and help to remain focused. It is a supercharger that keeps you light and agile both in body and mind. Starting the day with Bulletproof

Coffee ensures that your next stop for food would be late lunch. Does it not sound really special?

How to prepare it?

It's easy and simple like brewing any other coffee. Use the right recipe and you get Bulletproof Coffee in a few simple steps.

Ingredients:

➢ XCT oil or Brain Octane – 1 to 2 tablespoons. These are specially prepared oils (without flavor) which are 6 times and 18 times stronger than coconut oil.

➢ Unsalted grass-fed butter – 1to 2 tablespoons

➢ Hot brewed with Bulletproof Coffee beans - 1 to 2 cups (250 to 500 ml)

Directions:

✓ Brew Bulletproof Coffee beans as you normally would.

✓ Pre-heat the blender with boiling water.

✓ Drain the water from the blender and add butter, the brewed coffee and Brain Octane or XCT oil. Blend vigorously until the top layer if foaming and frothy.

✓   Make it special for you by adding dark chocolate, vanilla, cinnamon or a sweetener like erythritol or Stevia and enjoy.

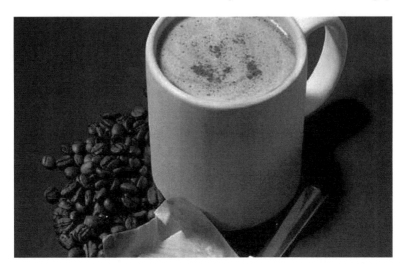

Is Bulletproof Coffee bad for you?

Is everything only good about Bulletproof Coffee? Well, how can that be? There cannot be anything called good or bad in absolute terms. Although the goodness of Bulletproof Coffee rules over the bad, it cannot be denied that there is a downside too. Let us find what is bad about Bulletproof Coffee and why is it bad for our health.

Reduction of total nutrient requirement

It is common for people to take three square meals every day – breakfast, lunch and dinner. Taking Bulletproof Coffee would effectively do away with the breakfast and the body's requirement of daily essential nutrients will have to come from lunch and dinner only. This means, you are falling short of total nutrients that your body needs. But the quantity of essential nutrients is very low in Bulletproof Coffee because XCT oil or Brain Octane are processed and refined fats that does not contain any essential nutrients but only 100% calories. Replacing the breakfast will obviously reduce your nutrient intake considerably that can be detrimental for your health.

High dose of healthy saturated fats

There is no doubt that the myth about the ill effects of saturated fats has been debunked and its healthy aspects have been put to good use in Bulletproof Coffee. It is now proved that saturated fat is not the cause of heart disease. But the question is – how much of saturated fat is safe for consumption?

It has been found that nutrients are safe and healthy when consumed in reasonable amounts. Excess consumption has shown bad effects. The amount of nutrients available from natural resources like fructose in fibrous fruits is good when consumed with the fruit but taking large doses of fructose from refined sugars can have alarming consequences.

The studies that have been conducted were based on normal intake of saturated fat, whereas its amount in Bulletproof Coffee is of course much higher than normal. When you take Bulletproof Coffee, you are eating saturated fat as a meal whereas saturated fat is supposed to be taken with a meal. As it is yet to be ascertained what amount of healthy fat is good for daily consumption, the consequences of overeating saturated fat can pose serious problems.

Increases cholesterol levels

Even if you have ensured a low carb diet with Bulletproof Coffee, you risk increasing the levels of LDL cholesterol (bad cholesterol) and effectively the total cholesterol as found in some studies. The risk of heart disease is obviously increased.

Difficult to sustain

There is no doubt that Bulletproof Coffee is one of the extreme diets that can make you shed considerable amount of body fat very rapidly. But the problem that you might face is in sticking to it in the long run. This has been the prime reason why extreme diets tend to fail.

You can weigh the benefits of Bulletproof Coffee and if you find it beneficial for your well being and health it is worthwhile to include Bulletproof Coffee in your diet plan.

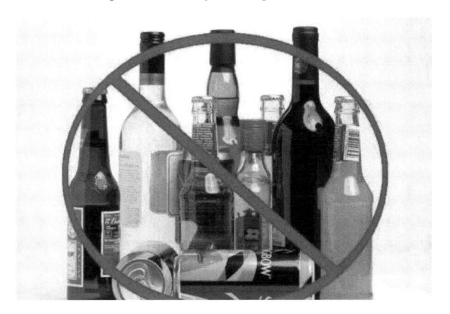

III. Bulletproof Diet and Alcohol Intake

When you decide to embark on Bulletproof diet it can be assumed that you want to cut down fat, be more energetic and focused while you also keep a check on your hunger. You set your eyes on calories and shun carbohydrates. But what about taking alcohol when you are on Bulletproof diet? One thing is clear that alcohol and Bulletproof diet does not go hand in hand simply because alcohol contains carbohydrates which are strictly prohibited by Bulletproof diet.

But does that mean that you have to abstain from partying in order to keep alcohol at bay? If you are on Bulletproof diet and also consume alcohol, then the body would prefer to burn alcohol rather than choosing all other nutrients that you consume. This would definitely defeat your purpose of taking up Bulletproof diet regimen as alcohol will decelerate the process of fat reduction by the conversion of free fatty acids to ketones. Keeping away from alcohol can be a very difficult proposition that might de-motivate you in pursuing Bulletproof diet.

But things are not as gloomy as you feel. There are ways of continuing with both alcohol and Bulletproof diet without compromising your health and fitness needs. The secret lies in making the right choice of alcohol that are high on calories but have negligible carbohydrate content. Select such alcohol that does not conflict with Bulletproof diet. Move over from light drinks that have high carbohydrate content and take up hard drinks in moderate quantities.

Drinks to avoid

Drinks that are high in carbohydrates should be avoided at all cost.

- Cocktails

- Beer

- Flavored liquor

- Mixers

- Wine

Drinks you can take

Here is a list of hard liquors that are free from carbohydrates but rich in calories that can be taken along with Bulletproof diet. The values of calories have been calculated per 1.5 oz. serving.

- Whiskey -105

- Gin - 102

- Vodka - 96

- Rum - 92

- Tequila – 96

Set your limits of alcohol intake because the level of ketosis in your body can be deepened by alcohol. It is also well known that liver metabolism is affected by alcohol that results in producing more ketones with higher alcohol intake. Alcohol is converted to a triglyceride that facilitates production of ketones.

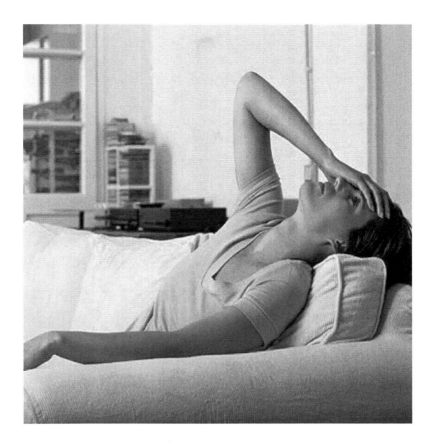

Curing Hangover

Now that you know what to drink you must also be concerned about hangover associated with alcohol. Here are some tips that can help you to cure hangover.

- Take a capsule each of Vitamin C and Unfair Advantage. This blocks the conversion of alcohol into aldehydes that causes hangover.

- Just before or after you consume a shot of drinks, make sure that you drink plenty of water. The more your body is hydrated, more easily the toxins will be diluted with water so that they become less harmful for your body.

- At the end of your drinking session, take 4 capsules of Activated charcoal.

- Begin and end your drinking session by taking Alpha Lipoic Acid or Vitamin B1 or N-Acetyl Ceistine. These facilitate fast absorption.

If you take the first step only then you will surely overcome hangover effects, but completing all the steps would ensure that you feel even much better than any other normal day.

IV. Yummy Recipes to Make Your Mouth Water

Here are some recipes that are easy to prepare and promises delicious serving while keeping up to the standards of Bulletproof diet. These dishes will not only satiate your appetite but will ensure that you are attuned to one of the healthiest eating habits that always keep you fit as a fiddle. Take a plunge into the world of some amazing recipes that will set your imagination on fire.

Breakfast Recipes

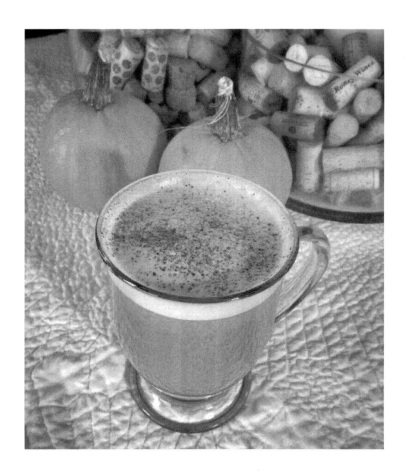

1. Bulletproof Pumpkin Spice Un-Latte

Ingredients (for 4-6 cups):

- Coconut milk unsweetened with full fat - 11/4 cup (canned coconut milk can be used)

- XCT oil or Brain octane oil - 3 tablespoons

- Blend of Stevia/Erythritol (maple syrup or raw honey will also do) - 2 tablespoons

- Organic pumpkin puree - 3 tablespoons

- Pumpkin pie spice – 1 teaspoon

- Unsalted butter (grass fed) – 1 tablespoon

- Bulletproof vanilla - ½ teaspoon

You are at liberty to add raw whipped cream 2 tablespoons on top or a tablespoon organic maple syrup.

Directions:

1. Mix all the ingredients in a saucepan.

2. Simmer over medium heat for about five minutes and stir well to ensure even blending of oils and spices.

3. Take 2 ½ cups of strongly brewed Bulletproof coffee in a blender and add the mixture of pumpkin and spice from the saucepan. Blend for half a minute on high till frothy and creamy. A hand blender may also be used for blending in saucepan.

4.   Top it up with cream or whipped cream to make it special if you want.

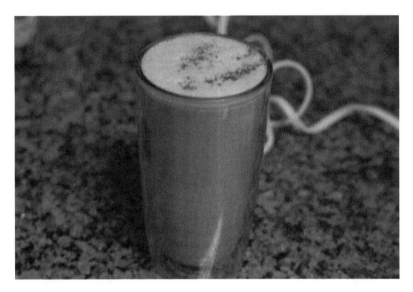

2. Bulletproof coffee

Ingredients (Single serving):

*   Bulletproof coffee beans – 2 ½ tablespoons heaped

*   Filtered water - 8 to 12 oz (1cup)

*   Brain octane – 1-2 tablespoons

*   Unsalted grass-fed butter or ghee – 1-2 tablespoons

You may add rice malt syrup, honey or stevia as sweetener.

Directions:

1. Brew a cup of coffee with filtered water that has just started boiling.

2. Mix the ingredients in a blender (that is pre-heated with hot water) till it develops froth like foamy latte.

The wonder drink is now ready for you to enjoy.

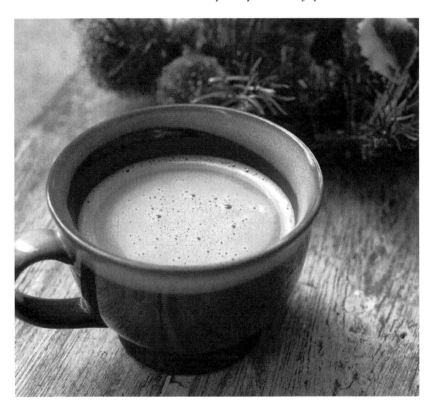

3. Bulletproof hot chocolate

Ingredients (Single serving):

- Coconut or almond milk – 1 cup (8-12 oz)

- Brain octane oil or coconut oil 1 ½ tablespoon

- Grass-fed butter or ghee or coconut oil mixed with ghee – 1 ½ tablespoon

- Cocoa/Cacao powder – 2 tablespoon

- Collagen powder – 1-2 tablespoon

- Sweetener (honey or maple syrup) – 1-2 tablespoon

Very small amount of vanilla extract and a thrifty sprinkling of cinnamon might be preferred by some people.

Directions:

1. Heat pot of coconut oil and butter together with milk till it melts.

2. The molten mass along with the other ingredients is blended at high speed in a blender for about 10-15 seconds.

3. Pour the blended mixture in a cup and savor its energizing effect.

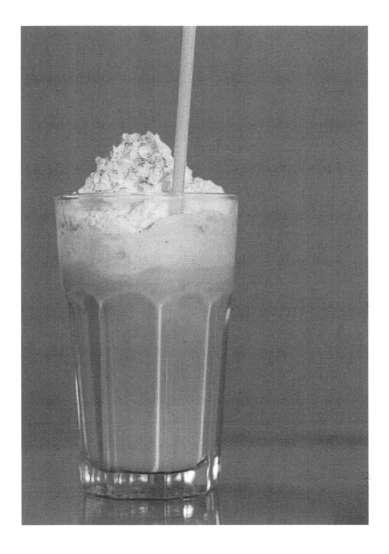

4. Bulletproof Coffee Shake

Ingredients (one serving of 3 cups):

- Organic coffee fresh brewed – 2 cups

- MCT oil – 1 tablespoon

- Organic coconut oil – 1 tablespoon

- Butter oil high vitamin – 1 teaspoon

- Grass-fed butter unsalted – 1-2 tablespoons

- Chocolate powder, raw organic – 1 ½ tablespoon

- Upgraded vanilla - ¼ teaspoon

- Organic cinnamon (ground) - ½ teaspoon

- Grass-fed Whey upgraded – 2-4 tablespoons

- Ice – 1-2 cups

Directions:

1. Leaving aside whey protein and ice, all other ingredients are blended.

2. Add ice to the mixture and blend

3. Add the upgraded whey (grass fed) and blend again but very briefly.

The lovable stuff is ready for serving.

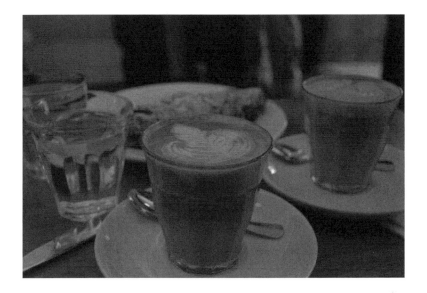

5. Bulletproof luscious Latte

Ingredients (single serving):

- Brewed Black coffee – 1 cup

- Virgin Coconut oil organic and unrefined – 1 tablespoon

- Vanilla extract – 1 teaspoon

- Cinnamon – a little more than a pinch

- Nutmeg – a dash of it

Directions:

1. Brew the coffee

2. Mix the coffee with coconut oil, vanilla extract and cinnamon in a blender

Pour it in a cup and start your healthy morning in great taste.

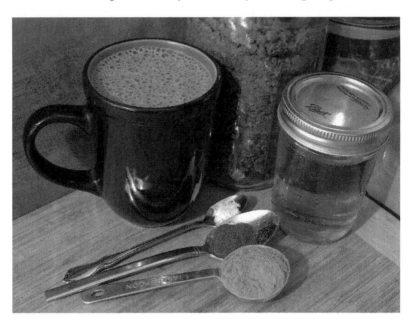

6. Bulletproof hot Chaga chocolate

Ingredients (single serving):

- Decoction of harvested Chaga in spring water   - 12 oz (1 cup)

- Organic cacao powder (raw) – 2 tablespoons

- Organic grass-fed butter (raw) – 1 ½ table spoons

- Maple syrup – 1 ½ tablespoons

- Salt – 1 pinch

- Organic vanilla powder (raw) – 1 pinch

Directions:

1. Heat Chaga decoction till it starts simmering.

2. Mix all the ingredients to it and blend it in a blender for about 20 seconds.

The drink is ready to be served.

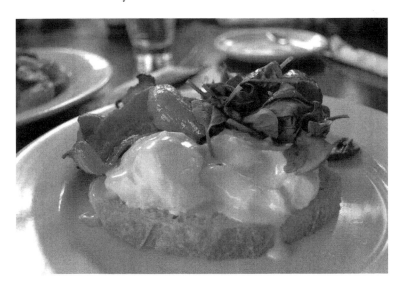

7. Bulletproof eggs Benedict with bacon and blender hollandaise sauce

Ingredients (single serving)

- Eggs yolks - 3

- Lemon juice - 1 to 2 tablespoon

- Salt – ¼ teaspoon

- Grass-fed butter – 8 tablespoons

Directions:

1. One tablespoon lemon juice along with yolks of egg and salt are mixed in blender and kept ready to be blended.

2. Butter is heated in a small saucepan at medium heat till it starts foaming.

3. Start blending the mixture of egg yolk for 2 seconds at top speed and while the blender is running, pour the hot butter in small droplets into the blender by removing its cover.

4. The sauce turns into thick cream when two-thirds of the butter has been added. Keep pouring the butter except for the milky residue.

5. Adjust seasonings as required by tasting at intervals.

The hollandaise sauce is ready to be taken with poached eggs and grilled bacon.

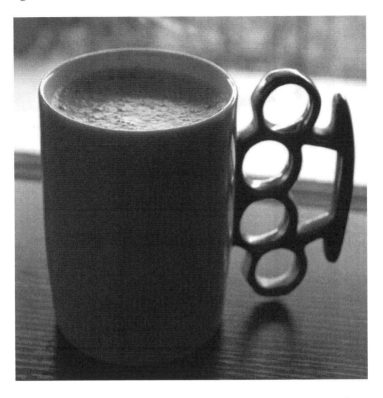

8. Bulletproof Maple Mocha

Ingredients (single serving):

- Hot coffee – 8oz (1 cup)
- Grass-fed butter – 1 teaspoon to ½ tablespoon

- Coconut Oil – 2 teaspoon to 2 tablespoon

- Coconut milk – 2 tablespoon

- Cocoa powder -1 tablespoon

- Maple syrup – ½ to 2 tablespoon

Directions:

Mix the ingredients in a blender till it is foamy and enjoy.

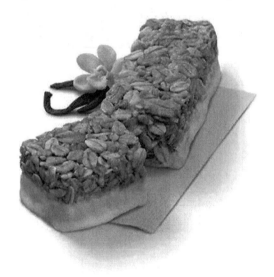

9. Good morning Granola with Orange Infused Yogurt

Ingredients (single serving of 12 cups):

- Rolled oats – 4 cups

- Unsweetened shredded coconut – 2 cups

- Sliced almonds – 2 cups

- Vegetable oil – ¾ cup

- Apricots (chopped and dried) – 1 ½ cups

- Honey - ¾ cup

- Calimyrna figs (chopped) – 1 cup

- Cranberries (dried) – 1 cup

- Cherries (dried) - 1 cup

- Walnuts or cashew toasted and chopped – 1 cup

- Orange infused yogurt (The recipe for this is given separately)

Directions:

1. Mix the oats, almonds and coconut in a large bowl and keep it ready for use.

2. Mix honey and oil in a small bowl and whisk for proper mixing.

3. Pour the honey and oil mixture on the oats, almonds, coconut mix and toss to coat.

4. Evenly spread out the mixture in a jelly roll pan.

5. Bake the granola for about 45 to 55 minutes at 225 degrees in an oven.

6. After 25 minutes, stir the mixture and again spread it evenly by means of a wooden spoon.

7. Rotate the pan and keep it in the oven for another half an hour or less so that the granola is toasted lightly.

8. Take out the granola from the oven and leave it in the pan for overnight cooling.

9. The morning after put the granola in a big bowl by breaking up the mass.

10. Add dried fruits like walnuts or cashews and mix by stirring.

The granola is ready to be served with Orange Infused Yogurt.

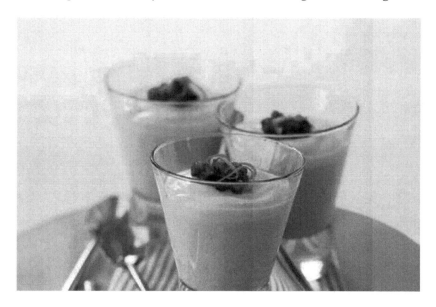

10. Good Orange Infused Yogurt

Ingredients:

- Organic whole milk yogurt – 1 quart

- Orange zest – 1 tablespoon

- Juiced Orange (preferably blood orange)

Directions:

1. Take a wire mesh strainer and line it with 2 layers of paper towels or 3 to 4 layers of cheese cloth.

2. Place the strainer on a bowl but ensure that there is a gap of at least 2 to 3 inches between the bowl and the strainer bottom.

3. Pour the yogurt in the strainer, cover it with a dishtowel and refrigerate and leave it overnight or at least 2 to 3 hours for draining.

4. After draining is completed, pour the yogurt in a bowl and remove the liner of the strainer.

5. Stir the yogurt after add juice and orange zest it.

The yogurt is ready to be served with Good Morning Granola.

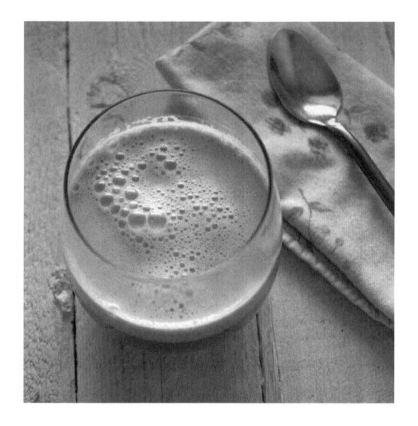

11. Bulletproof Chai

Ingredients (single serving for 1-2):

- Organic black tea, strong brewed – 2 cups

- Organic coconut oil – 1 tablespoon

- Grass-fed butter - 1 tablespoon

- Ground ginger – ¼ teaspoon

- Ground cinnamon – ¼ cup

- Honey – 1 teaspoon or stevia – a few drops

Directions:

1. Make a frothy emulsion of the ingredients by blending in a blender at high speed.

2. The drink is ready to be served.

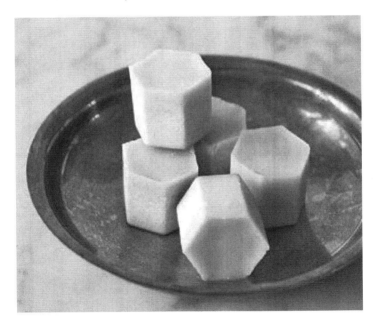

12. Bulletproof Coffee Drops

Ingredients (single serving):

- Grass-fed unsalted butter – ½ stick

- MCT or coconut oil – ½ cup

- Cinnamon – ½ teaspoon

- Sea salt – ¼ teaspoon

Directions:

1. Mix melted coconut oil with butter, cinnamon and sea salt.

2. Whisk it and then pour into an ice cube tray.

3. After freezing, remove the drops and store it in a glass container in the fridge.

The drops are ready for use whenever you like.

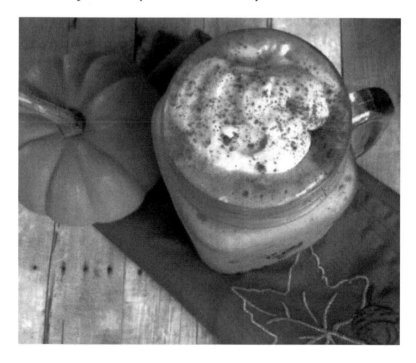

13. Bulletproof Pumpkin Frappuccino

Ingredients (single serving for 1 large or 2 small Frappuccino)

- Cold coffee – 1 ½ cups

- Pumpkin puree – ¼ cup

- Vanilla almond milk (unsweetened) – 1 ¼ cups

- Sweetener Splenda (or others) – 4 packets

- Cloves – ¼ teaspoon

- Cinnamon (ground) – 1 teaspoon

- Nutmeg (ground) – ¼ teaspoon

- Heavy cream may be used if you like.

Directions:

1. Make cold coffee by refrigerating brewed coffee overnight.

2. Take the pumpkin, milk, sweetener, cloves, cinnamon and nutmeg in a small bowl and whisk to mix properly.

3. Pour the mixture into ice trays and put it in a refrigerator for making frozen cubes.

4. Put the frozen cubes in a food processor or blender and blend at high speed until icy and smooth.

5. Add as much cream as you like to get the texture you desire.

6. Use whipped cream as topping if you want.

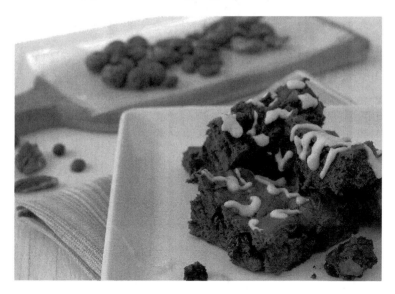

14. Blueberry Espresso Brownies

Ingredients (single serving for 12):

- Coconut cream concentrate (melted) – 1 cup

- Eggs – 3

- Blueberries – 1 cup

- Raw organic honey – ½ cup

- Organic Cocoa powder – ¼ cup

- Pecans (crushed) – 1 cup

- Ground coffee (your choice) – 1 tablespoon

- Cinnamon – 1 tablespoon

- Baking soda – ½ teaspoon

- Vanilla extract – 2 teaspoons

- Sea salt - ¼ teaspoon

Directions:

1. Begin by preheating your oven to 325 degrees Fahrenheit.

2. Take all the ingredients barring the blueberries in a mixing bowl.

3. Blend the ingredients well in a mixer – stand mixer or hand mixer.

4. Fold in the blueberries using your hand taking care to avoid crushing them.

5. Grease a baking dish of size 9 by 13 with coconut oil and pour the batter into it. You can also use mini muffin pans.

6. Bake it in the oven for half an hour approximately while doing the toothpick test just before completion to gauge how much baking is left to be done.

7. Take out from the oven and cool.

8. After cooling, spread some coconut cream concentrate over the brownies.

Just cut it and enjoy.

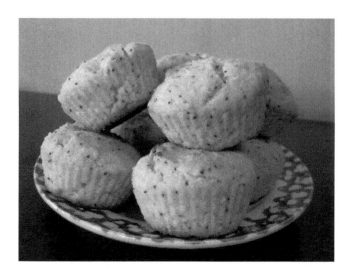

15. Lemon Poppy seed muffins (with coconut flour)

Ingredients (single serving for 8):

- Coconut flour – ½ cup

- Baking soda – ¼ teaspoon

- Salt – ½ teaspoon

- Eggs – 4

- Xantham gum– ½ teaspoon (optional)

- Honey – ½ cup

- Oil – 1/3 cup

- Poppy seeds – 1 tablespoon

- Vanilla – 1 tablespoon

- Juice of whole lemon (medium) – 1

- Lemon Zest from medium lemon – 1 tablespoon

Directions:

1. Start by preheating the oven to 350 degree Fahrenheit.

2. Mix coconut flour, baking soda, salt, poppy seeds and Xantham gum in a large bowl.

3. Mix honey eggs, vanilla, oil, lemon juice and lemon zest in a medium bowl. Grate lemon in a cheese grater on the finer side to obtain lemon zest.

4. Combine the wet and dry ingredients so that they mix well.

5. Pour the batter in silicone cups or muffin tins to fill them up to three quarter of volume.

6. Bake for 12 minutes if you are using small muffins and for larger muffins it should take15 to 18 minutes for baking. However, you will have to rely on the toothpick test to ascertain the exact time for baking.

7. Take out from the oven, cool it and serve.

Lunch recipes

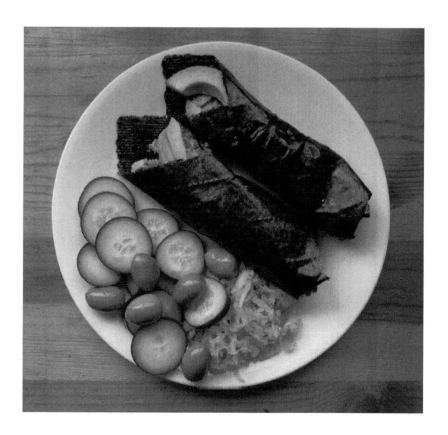

1. Avocado and salmon " Not Sushi"

Ingredients (single serving):

- Hass Avocado – 1

- Wild sockeye salmon smoked cold – 4 oz

Directions:

1. Cut the salmon and avocado into four slices each. The avocado slices should be about ¼ inch thick.

2. Take each salmon slice and wrap it with avocado.

3. Sprinkle some salt on it.

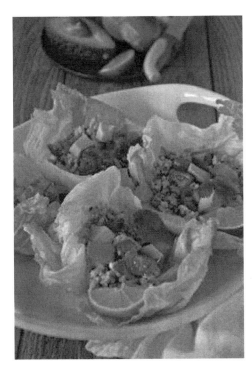

2. Taco Salad

The recipe consists of Taco mix, Avocado dressing and Salad.

Taco Mix

Ingredients (4 serving):

- Grass-fed Organic fatty ground feed beef – 1 lb

- Fresh lime (squeezed) – ½

- Grass-fed butter unsalted or ghee – 2 tablespoon

- Dried oregano – 1 teaspoon

- Cayenne powder – 1 tablespoon

- Sea salt – according to your taste

Avocado dressing

- Avocado – 2

- Apple cider vinegar – ¼ cup

- MCT oil – ¼ cup

- Sliced cucumber – 4 cups

- Fresh lemon juice – ¼ cup

- Fresh cilantro (chopped) – 1 cup

- Sea salt – according to your taste

- Spring onions – 4 (optional)

Salad

- Spring lettuce – 1 cup

- Carrots (shredded) – 2

- Red cabbage (shredded) – ¼ cup

- Avocado sliced – ½

- Cucumber sliced – 1

Directions:

1. Sauté beef in a medium pan until it is thoroughly cooked and then drain excess fat. Add ghee or butter, oregano, cayenne powder, lime juice and salt. Set aside after removing from heat.

2. Mix ingredients of salad and make it into four plates after topping with beef mixture.

3. Put the dressing ingredients in a blender and blend to make it creamy and smooth.

4. Drizzle it over salad

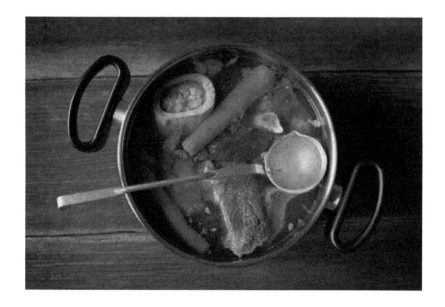

3. Bulletproof Bone Broth

Ingredients (single serving):

- Medium Carrot, peeled and cut into chunks (peeled) – 3

- Beef marrow bones (assorted) – 2 ½ pounds

- Stalk Celery, peeled and cut into chunks – 3

- Upgraded Collagen – 1 cup per liter of broth (optional)

- Apple cider vinegar - 1 to 2 tablespoons

- Fresh bouquet gami (rosemary, sage, fresh oregano or thyme – as you like) – 1

- Sea salt – according to your taste

Directions:

1. Sauté the celery and carrots lightly in a large stockpot for a few minutes till it turns translucent.

2. Add the bouquet gami and beef bones and cover with water to which you can add apple cider vinegar to extract the nutrients from the bones. For 8 to 14 hours, simmer on low heat but avoid boiling.

3. Strain out the vegetables and remove the bones after the broth attains the desired flavor and colour.

4. Add Collagen (if you are using) and stir well till it dissolves.

5. Add salt.

The broth is ready to serve or you can preserve it by storing in mason jars and freezing it.

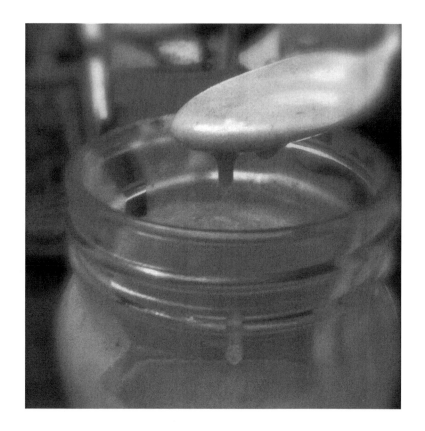

4. Honey Mustard Vinaigrette

Ingredients (single serving):

- Extra Virgin olive oil – 1/8 cup

- Apple cider vinegar – ¼ cup

- Organic mustard – 3 tablespoon

- Brain Octane – 1/8 cup

- Xylitol or raw honey- 2 tablespoon

Directions:

Blend the ingredients to get the food of your choice.

5. **Bulletproof Salad Dressing**

Ingredients (single serving):

- Yolks of egg-2 or Avocado – ½

- Brain Octane oil – 3 tablespoon

- Coconut Oil – 2 tablespoon (optional)

- Cucumber (medium) – 1/3

- Apple cider vinegar – 2 tablespoon

- Sea salt – as per your taste

- Stevia or Xylitol – 1 pinch

- Fresh oregano, cilantro or pepper (spicy or sweet)

Directions:

Get a salad dressing that is creamy and thick by proper blending of the ingredients.

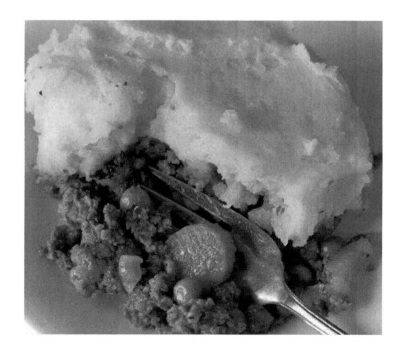

6. Bulletproof Shepherd's Pie

The dish consists of cooking ground beef, carrots, red cabbage and mashed cauliflower and then layered upon one another and cooked in an oven.

Beef layer - bottom

Ingredients (6 servings):

- Grass-fed Angus ground beef – 1 pound

- Coconut flour – 1 tablespoon

- Vegetable stock – ½ cup (optional for thickening gravy)

Cabbage layer – Middle

- Bacon grease – 1 to 2 tablespoon

- Grass-fed Butter – 1 tablespoon

- Head of cabbage (shredded) – less than ¼

- Carrots (diced) – 2

- Partly sliced three leaks white

- Mustard – 1 tablespoon

- Apple cider vinegar – ¼ cup

Mashed cauliflower – top

- Cauliflower – 1 head

- Chopped thyme – 1 bunch

- Chopped chives – 1 bunch

- Salt – as required

Directions:

Beef layer

Mix ½ cup water with ground beef and cook on medium to low heat.

1. Break open cayenne pepper capsules to add a dash of it, if you like.

2. Transfer beef to baking dish.

3. If you want gravy then mix ½ tablespoon coconut flour to half cup of vegetable stock to the cooking pan containing beef.

4. Keep stirring and as soon as it thickens add again half spoon coconut flour to it for speedy thickening.

Cabbage layer

1. Add butter and bacon grease in the pan and heat (medium).

2. Put in the leaks and cook for few minutes.

3. Add cabbage and carrots.

4. Cook for 10 to 15 minutes on medium heat to low heat after adding apple cider vinegar.

5. Spread it on top of the beef kept in the baking dish.

Mashed cauliflower

1. Steam the chopped cauliflower to make it tender.

2. Take the steamed cauliflower in a blender or food processor, add butter and blend it.

3. Spread the mashed cauliflower on the cabbage layer and sprinkle some quantity of fresh thyme on the top.

4. Make the mashed cauliflower a bit crispy by baking for 15 minutes at 350 degree Fahrenheit.

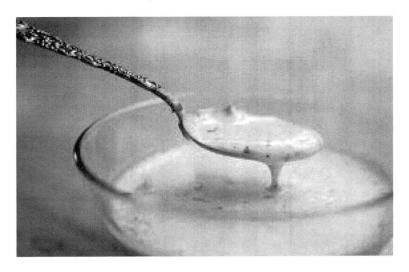

7. Bulletproof Ranch Dressing

This recipe includes Bulletproof Mayonnaise, the recipe of which has been given separately.

Ingredients (single serving):

*   Fresh Dill (chopped) – 2 tablespoon

*   Bulletproof Mayonnaise – 1 cup

*   Apple cider vinegar – 1 tablespoon

*   2 Cloves and garlic minced and mixed with sea salt

- Pepper and salt

Directions:

Blend the ingredients and then chill for a few hours to make it ready for serving.

Bulletproof Mayonnaise

- Egg (large) – 1

- Brain Octane – ¼ cup

- Extra light Olive Oil – ¾ cup

- Salt – 1 pinch

- Lime or lemon juice (fresh squeezed) – 2 to 3 teaspoons

Directions:

1. Take all the ingredients in a container and allow the egg to settle at the bottom of the container.

2. Then blend with an immersion blender till you get the desired consistency of mayo.

3. For emulsification, you can add soy lecithin, avocado or another egg yolk.

4. Use fresh herbs to add flavor.

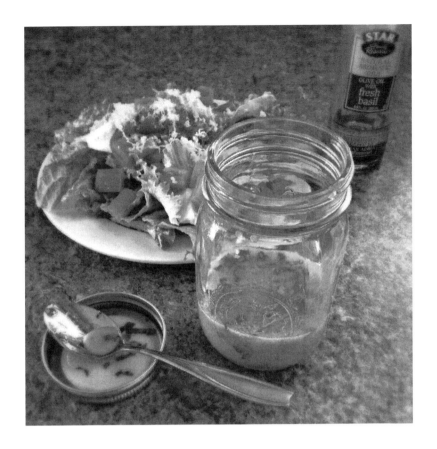

8. Creamy Basil Vinaigrette

Ingredients (single serving):

- Avocado – ½

- Brain Octane – 2 tablespoon

- Extra Virgin olive Oil – ¼ cup

- Apple cider vinegar -1/4 cup

- Basil leaves – a small handful

Directions:

Do a perfect blending of the ingredients to prepare the delicacy.

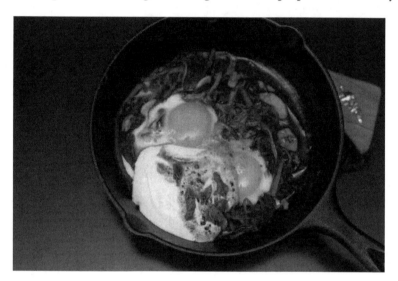

9. Poached eggs with Saluted greens

Ingredients (single serving):

- Collards, kale or chard – 2 to 3 cups

- Raw almonds or cashews (sliced) – 2 tablespoon

- Grass-fed unsalted butter or ghee – 2 tablespoon

- Poached eggs – 2

- Sea salt

Directions:

1. Cook the greens in a medium frying pan in water (about an inch of water will do) to make it tender.

2. After draining the water, add ghee or butter and toss. The greens will get a coated.

3. Add nuts and salt after removing from the heat and keep it aside.

4. Top eggs with nuts and greens for serving.

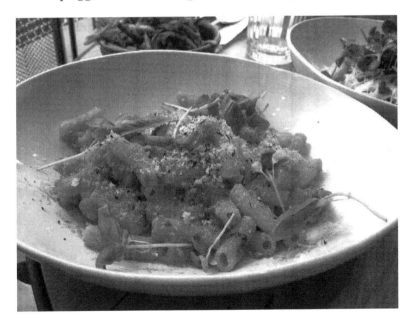

10. Penne all' Arrabbiata

Ingredients (4 servings):

- Penne Pasta (dried) – 1 pound

- Arrabiatta sauce – 2-3 cups (recipe is given below)

- Parmigiano-Reggiano cheese (grated) – ½ cup

- Parsley (chopped) - 3 tablespoons

Directions:

1. Take a large pot and cook the penne in rapidly boiling water to which salt has been added in order to prevent sticking.

2. The pasta can be undercooked, as it's cooking gets completed in the presence of sauce.

3. Warm Arrabbiata sauce (2 to 3 cups) in a skillet or sauté pan.

4. Add the cooked pasted (after draining well) to Arrabbiata sauce and toss it gently with the sauce for good coating.

5. Toss again after adding 3 tablespoons parsley.

6. Use grated cheese for topping each serving.

Arrabbiata Sauce

Ingredients

- Fresh ripe tomatoes – 1 to 1 ½ pounds

- Garlic cloves (large) – 4

- Olive oil – 3 to 4 tablespoons

- Fresh Serrano chili pepper (chopped) – 1 OR Red pepper flakes - ½ teaspoon

- Fresh basil leaves (shredded) – a few (optional)

Directions:

1. Core the fresh tomatoes and quarter them and puree them in a blender or food processor and set aside.

2. Heat the olive oil over medium heat in a heavy sauce pan and add garlic when the oil is hot and about to sizzle. Cook the garlic for one or two minutes while stirring till you get the aroma. But do not allow the garlic to turn brown.

3. Add the fresh chili or pepper flakes, keep stirring and add the tomatoes.

4. Boil the sauce, lower the heat and leave it uncovered for simmering for about 45 minutes or till the time the sauce gets thick and reduces in volume.

5. Towards the end of cooking, add salt and pepper for seasoning and add basil leaves if you wish.

You get about 3 ½ cups sauce from the above.

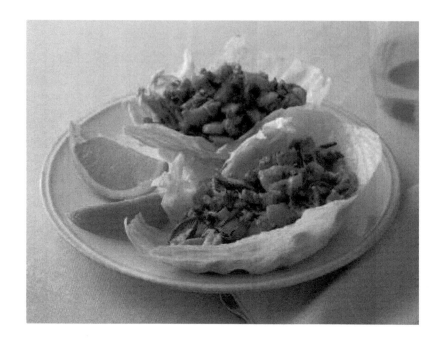

11. Chinese Lettuce Wrap

Ingredients (single serving):

- Carrots – 2-3

- Squash – 1

- Cucumber (large) – 1

- Zucchini – 1

- Mushroom – 1 to 2 cups

- Olive oil – ½ pound

- Grass-fed ground beef
- ~~Soy Sauce~~ *coconut aminos*
- Chinese cooking alcohol
- Cloves of garlic - 4 to 5
- Green onion – 1
- Iceberg lettuce

Directions:

1. Cut all the vegetables into small dice like cubes.

2. Cook the beef in 2 spoons of olive oil that is heated in a pan. Keep stirring slowly till the beef is cooked. Take out the beef from the pan when done and keep it aside.

3. Now add garlic and green onion to the pan followed by carrots. Cook for 3 to 4 minutes as you keep stirring.

4. For flavoring, add Chinese alcohol (4 to 5 spoons).

5. Add the remaining vegetables and soy sauce and some water (½ cup) if it is too dry. Then cook for 4 to 5 minutes.

6. Now add beef and wait for a minute or two by when all the vegetables get cooked.

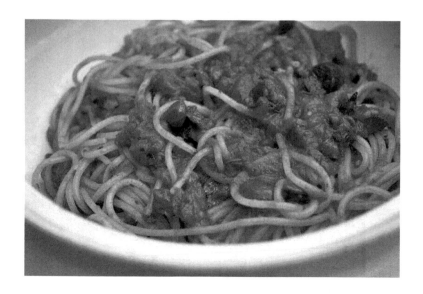

12. Penne alla Puttanesca

Ingredients (4 servings):

- Anchovy fillets (chopped) – 3 to 4

- Olive oil – 2 tablespoons

- Capers (chopped) – 1 tablespoon

- Clove garlic – 1

- Oil cured olives or 12 drained Kalamata (large but sliced into quarter)

- Arrabbiata sauce – 2 to 3 cups

- White wine (dry) ¼ cup

- Cooked Penne pasta – 1 pound

Directions:

1. Take anchovies and garlic in a skillet or sauté pan and heat with olive oil at medium heat while stirring until you find that the anchovies have melted.

2. Add the olives, capers and wine at simmering heat for 2 minutes approximately.

3. Now add Arrabbiata sauce (recipe given earlier) and allow 5 minutes simmering at low heat.

4. Add cooked Penne pasta and toss with sauce until a good coating is done.

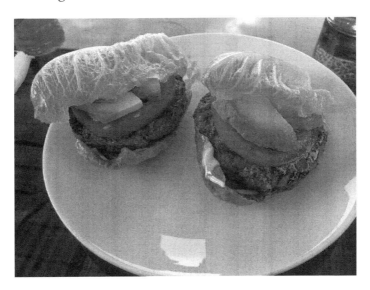

13. Lettuce Wrap grass-fed Burger

Ingredients (Single serving):

- Grass-fed ground beef

- Iceberg lettuce

- Avocados – 2

- Tomato – ½

- Cloves of garlic – 4-5

Directions:

1. Make burger patties using your own method and grill to make it ready to use.

2. Mix diced up garlic, tomato and avocados along with salt in a bowl.

3. Wrap the ingredients with lettuce. For better taste you can lightly sauté the lettuce before serving.

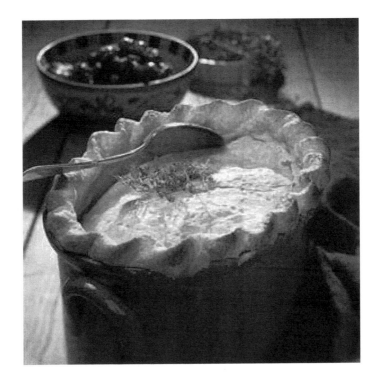

14. Chicken Pot pie – The Sequel

Pot Pie

Ingredients (single serving):

- Diced bacon – 3 slices

- Carrot (diced) – 1

- Onion (chopped) – 1

- Clove garlic (crushed) – 1

- Stalk Celery (diced) – 1

- Cut green beans – 1 cup

- Canned coconut milk – 1 ¼ oz.

- Chicken stock – 1 cup

- Pepper – ½ teaspoon

- Salt – 1 teaspoon

- Arrowroot – 2 tablespoon

- Cooked chicken (chopped) – 2 cups

Directions:

1. Cook bacon in a medium size pot till it is crispy.

2. After adding celery, carrot, garlic and onion cook for 5 minutes.

3. Add coconut milk, chicken stock, pepper, salt, poultry seasoning, chicken and green beans and make it boil.

4. Reduce the heat to simmer and mix one tablespoon arrowroot. Keep stirring until it dissolves.

5. Make it thick by simmering a little more.

6. Pour into baking dish of size 8x12.

Dough

Ingredients

- Tapioca flour – 1 cup

- Baking soda – ¼ teaspoon

- Coconut flour – 1/4cup

- Cream of tartar – ½ teaspoon

- Boiling water – ½ cup

- Coconut oil or butter – 3 tablespoon

- Salt – ½ teaspoon

Directions:

1. Form crumbles of the dry ingredients by mixing butter to it.

2. Moisten the dry ingredients with hot water.

3. Form ball and convert these to rectangular flats.

4. Place the rectangular flats upon pot pie ingredients and bake for 10 minutes at 400 degrees Fahrenheit.

Dinner Recipes

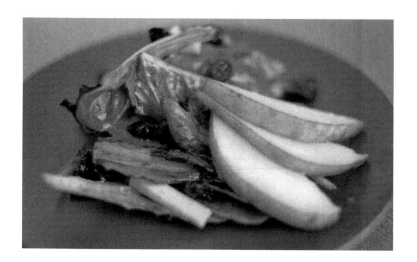

1. Pear Salad with lemon Rosemary Vinaigrette and chocolate drizzle

Salad Base

Ingredients (2 servings):

- Organic baby greens (mixed) – 3 cups
- Sliced shallot (small) – 1

Directions:

Set aside the mixture of the ingredients taken in a salad bowl.

Lemon Rosemary Vinaigrette dressing

Ingredients

- Upgraded XCT oil – ½ cup

- Fresh rosemary (chopped) – 1 tablespoon

- Juiced lemon – ½

- Pear slice (peeled) size ¼" – 1

- Garlic clove (crushed) – 1

- Dijon mustard – 1/8 teaspoon

- Fresh pepper (ground)

- Himalayan salt

Directions:

Combine the ingredients and smoothen in a blender. Keep it aside.

Chocolate pear drizzle

Ingredients

- Organic honey raw – 1 teaspoon

- Pear with skin (sliced) – 1

- Chocolate – ½ oz.

- Fresh thyme (chopped) – 1 tablespoon

- Cayenne pepper – 1 to 2 pinches

- Goat cheese (crumbled)- ¼ cup

- Fresh rosemary (chopped finely) – ¼ teaspoon

Directions:

1. Preheating of oven to 350 degrees Fahrenheit is the first step.

2. Place the sliced pears on a cookie sheet lined with parchment paper.

3. Lightly sprinkle chopped thyme and honey on pears.

4. Bake in oven for 8 to 10 minutes until beginning to soften.

5. During this time, melt half ounce of chocolate (bulletproof) over medium heat in a saucepan.

6. Add rosemary and cayenne to the fully molten chocolate. Stir and then let it sit.

7. After the pears are baked, remove from oven and with the help of a spoon, give a light drizzle of molten chocolate sauce on it before setting it aside.

8. Toss salad with Rosemary/Lemon vinaigrette; give a topping of crumbled goat cheese and pears to complete the dish that is now ready to be served.

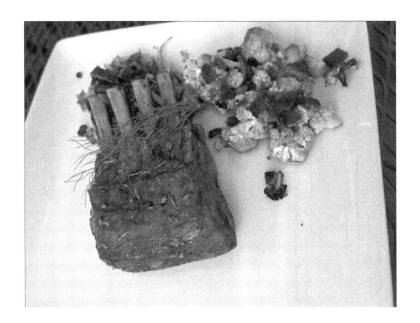

2. Roasted lamb Rack with cauliflower, celery and fennel

Ingredients (3 servings):

- American rack of lamb (grass-fed, organic, 8 chops) – 1 ½ pounds

- Fennel (sliced) – 2 cups

- Ghee – 1 tablespoon

- Celery (sliced) – 2 cups

- Oregano, thyme, sage (all chopped), rosemary sea salt and turmeric -1 tablespoon each

- Cauliflower (sliced) -2 cups

Directions:

1. Make the oven ready by preheating it to 350 degrees Fahrenheit.

2. Apply ghee on lamb and then score fat across diagonally.

3. Sprinkle salt and chopped herbs over lamb.

4. Take a roasting pan and place the vegetables in it. Lay lamb on to with fat side up.

5. Bake for about 45 minutes until the thickest part of lamb reaches 125 degrees Fahrenheit.

6. To crisp the skin, cook for approximately another 3 minutes, at low broil.

7. Pulled Pork Shoulder with Brussels Sprout

8. Pulled Pork Shoulder with Brussels Sprout

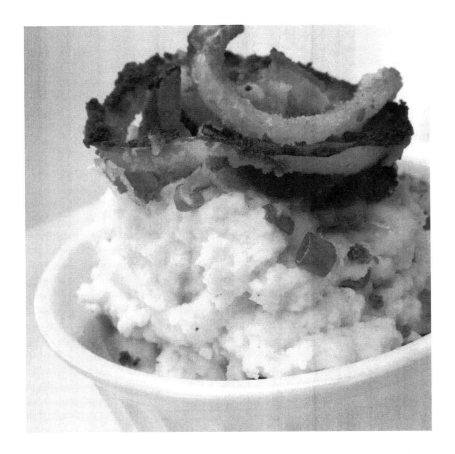

3. Cauliflower bacon Mash

Ingredients (2 to 4 servings):

- Cauliflower, large head (cut into florets) – 1

- Upgraded XCT oil – 2 tablespoons

- Grass-fed unsalted butter – 4 tablespoons

- Bacon (pastured, preservative free, medium low cooked, diced) – ½ pound

- Apple cider vinegar – ½ tablespoon

- Sea salt – as you desire

Directions:

1. Steam the cauliflower to make it tender and then drain.

2. Take ¾ cauliflowers and mix other ingredients to it leaving aside the bacon.

3. Add the bacon while stirring and pulse until chunks are formed.

4. Add bacon grease (1 to 2 tablespoons) at the time when you are cooking the bacon at low heat.

   The dish is ready to be served.

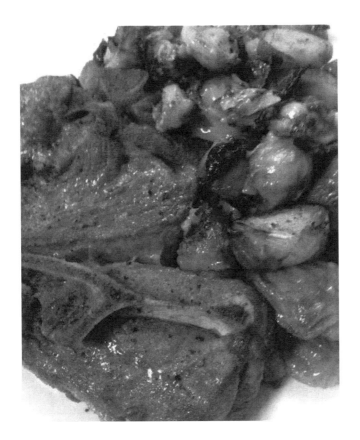

4. Pulled Pork Shoulder with Brussels Sprout

Ingredients (4 servings):

Pork preparation

- Pastured bacon, uncooked – 6 strips

- Oregano (dried) – 2 tablespoons

- Pastured pork shoulder – 4 lbs.

- Turmeric (ground) – 3 teaspoon

- Apple cider vinegar – ½ cup (optional)

- Xylitol – ½ cup (optional)

- Sea salt – as needed

Brussels Sprout preparation

- Brussels sprouts (cut into halves) -1 pound

- Sea salt – 2 teaspoons

- Turmeric (ground) – 2 teaspoons

- Grass-fed unsalted butter – 2 tablespoons

Directions:

1. Put the bacon strips in a slow cooker so that they are placed at the base.

2. Rub oregano, salt and turmeric on pork, place it upon the bacon and cook for about 14-16 hours.

3. Use a fork to shred meat.

4. To impart a tangy barbecue flavor (sweet and sour) mix drippings from slow cooker with apple cider vinegar and

xylitol in a pan and simmer at low heat for 5 minutes and you get the sauce that adds zing.

5.   Preheat oven to 300 degrees Fahrenheit.

6.   Take a baking pan, put the Brussels sprouts into it and coat with butter, turmeric and salt.

7.   Bake for about 30 minutes to 45 minutes.

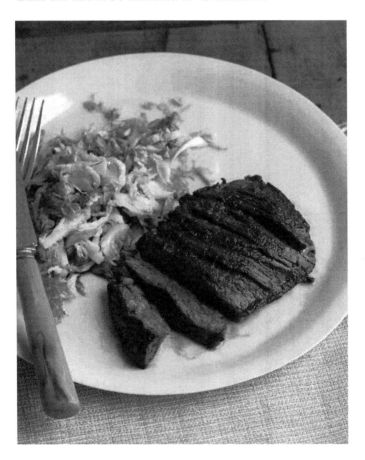

5. Bulletproof Roast with Brussels Sprouts

Ingredients (2 to 4 servings):

Meat

- Organic bottom sirloin or skirt steak (grass-fed) – 1 lb.

- Grass-fed unsalted butter – 3 tablespoons

- Upgraded XCT oil – 2 tablespoons

- Turmeric (ground) – 1 tablespoon

- Sea salt – 2 tablespoons

- Oregano (dried) – 1 teaspoon

- Apple cider vinegar – 1 ½ tablespoons

Brussels sprouts

- Halved Brussels sprouts – 1 lb.

- Sea salt – 2 teaspoons

- Grass-fed unsalted butter – 2 teaspoons

- Turmeric (ground) – 2 teaspoons

Directions:

1. Rub the meat with salt, oregano and turmeric.

2.	Place it in a slow cooker and add the upgraded XCT oil to it.

3.	Add butter, cook for 6-8 hours so that the meat becomes shred able.

4.	Add vinegar after cooking is completed.

The meat preparation is complete.

1.	Make the oven ready by preheating to 350 degrees Fahrenheit.

2.	Take the sprouts in a baking pan and add butter to it.

3.	Sprinkle turmeric and salt and bake for about 30-45 minutes.

The Brussels sprouts are ready to be served.

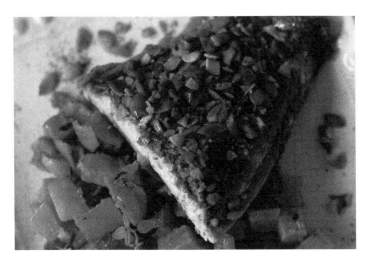

6. Baked Fish with Steamed butternut Squash

Ingredients (4 servings):

Fish preparation

- Tilapia fillets – 1 pound

- Vanilla powder – ¼ teaspoon

- Coffee beans (ground) – ¼ cup

- Turmeric (ground) – 1 tablespoon

- Oregano (dried) – 1 tablespoon

- Xylitol – 3 tablespoons

- Sea salt – 2 tablespoons

Squash preparation

- Butternut Squash cubes of 1 inch (seeded but peeled) – 1 medium

- MCT oil – 2 to 3 tablespoons

- Carrots cut into cubes of 1 inch (peeled) – 4 medium

- Spring onion (cut) – 4 pieces

- Apple cider vinegar – ½ tablespoon

- Grass-fed unsalted butter – 4 tablespoons

- Sea salt – according to taste

Directions:

1. Start by preheating the oven to 320 degrees Fahrenheit.

2. Mix vanilla powder, coffee beans, xylitol, salt, oregano and turmeric in a small bowl.

3. Rub the mixture over fish.

4. Place fish in a baking dish in single layer, put it in the middle rack of the oven and bake for about 10 minutes till it is oven thoroughly cooked.

5. Put the carrots and squash for steaming till tender.

6. Take it in a blender with other ingredients and blend well till you get the consistency like mashed potatoes.

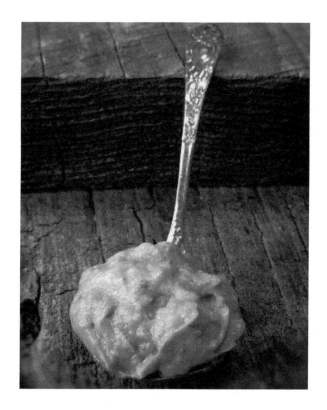

7. Guacamole (Bulletproof)

Ingredients (single serving):

- Haas Avocado (large and ripe) – 4

- Organic oregano (dried) – 1 tablespoon

- Upgraded XCT oil or Brain Octane – 2 to 4 tablespoons

- Apple cider vinegar – 1-3 teaspoon as per taste needs

- Himalayan salt – 2 teaspoons or as required.

Directions:

Use a hand blender to blend the ingredients until it turns creamy.
Add herbs of your choice jalapenos and cilantro as you stir.

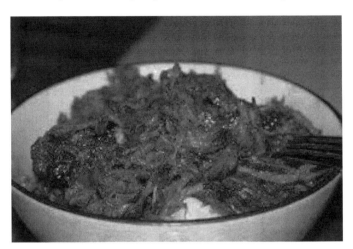

8. Sweet Crockpot pulled Pork

Ingredients (single serving):

- Brandy – 1/8 cup

- Bone in pork shoulder – 5 pounds

- Cinnamon – 1 teaspoon

- Sweet paprika -2 teaspoons

- Nutmeg – 1 teaspoon

- Sea salt -2 teaspoon

- Ginger – 1 teaspoon

- Garlic powder – ½ tablespoon

- Onion powder – ½ tablespoon

- Black pepper (ground) – ½ teaspoon

- Mustard (dry) – ½ tablespoon

Directions:

1. Leaving aside brandy and pork shoulder, mix all other ingredients in a small mixing bowl to obtain the spice rub.

2. Apply the spice rub over the meat so that it enters into all crevices that you see.

3. Wrap the spice laden meat in a plastic wrap (preferably double wrap and refrigerate for at least 3 hours. You can even leave it in the freezer for 3 days.

4. When done, unwrap it and place it in your crock pot while you add 1/8 cup water and the same amount of brandy to it.

5. Put the crock pot on low heat and cook for 8 to 10 hours until the meat becomes tender enough to be handled by fork.

6. Take out the roast to a cutting board, discarding the liquid in the crock pot.

7. Use your fingers or a fork to shred the meat.

8. Put back the shredded meat in the crock pot and toss with Raspberry BBQ sauce at low heat for about an hour until it is hot.

9. You have now got the delicacy that can be served and enjoyed.

Raspberry BBQ sauce

Ingredients: (makes for 3 cups):

• White Onion (minced) – 1

• Extra virgin olive oil – 4 tablespoons

• Homemade ketchup – ½ cup

• Jalapeno – 1 along with minced seeds

• Raw organic honey (melted) – 2 tablespoons

• Frozen raspberries – 4 cups

• Cayenne – ½ teaspoon

• Mustard (dry) – ½ teaspoon

Directions:

1. Heat some coconut oil at medium heat in a non stick sauce pan, add onions and jalapeno and leave it for 10 minutes for sweating.

2. Add mustard, honey, ketchup, and cayenne and keep heating till the mixture starts simmering.

3. Add the frozen raspberries and continue simmering for 15 minutes till mixing becomes uniform.

4. Cool the stuff and take it in a blender for smooth blending.

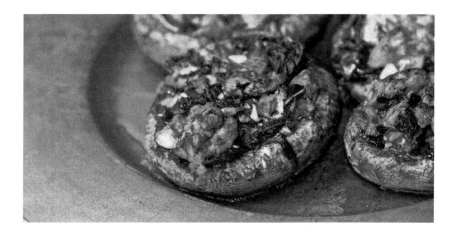

9. Giant Stuffed Mushrooms

Ingredients (single serving):

•   Portobello mushrooms (big) – 4 to 6

•   Italian pork sausage (spicy, casing removed) – 1 pound

- Grass-fed ground beef – 1 ½ pounds
- Celery stalks (dried) – 3
- Red onion (diced) – 1
- Green bell pepper (diced) – ½
- Paprika – 1 teaspoon
- Mushroom stems (diced)
- Basil (dried) – 2 tablespoons
- Cayenne pepper – ½ teaspoon to a few shakes
- Garlic cloves (crushed) – 6
- Tarragon – 1 tablespoon
- Salt – 1 pinch
- Egg (omega 3 enriched) – 1
- Black pepper – according to taste
- Coconut flour – ¼ cup
- Olive oil – ¼ cup

Directions:

1. Preheat the oven to 400 degrees Fahrenheit.

2. Wipe the mushrooms clean with moist paper towel but do not clean it under water, as it gets soggy. Use a spoon to

remove the feathery insides of the mushrooms, remove the stems and keep aside.

3.   Wipe olive oil on the outsides of the mushrooms and place it in a baking dish with cap down.

4.   Dice the celery stalks, onions, bell peppers and mushroom stems.

5.   Brown the ground beef and sausage in a large soup pot, add mushrooms, celery, onions and bell peppers and cook until the vegetables become tender.

6.   Take the mixture in a food processor and add egg, spices coconut flour and olive oil and process it until the mixture is chopped finely but take care that it is not mushy.

7.   Fill the mushrooms caps with the mixture of meat and vegetables.

8.   Use the preheated oven to cook the mushrooms till it turns bubbly and brown in about 20 minutes

You can serve this with steamed kale seasoned with garlic powder, lemon juice, freshly ground pepper and olive oil.

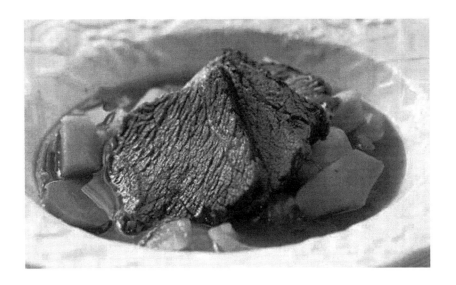

10. Primal Pot Roast

Ingredients:

- Paprika – 1 tablespoon

- Thyme (dried) – 1 teaspoon

- Rosemary (dried and crushed) – 1 teaspoon

- Black pepper (freshly ground) – 1 teaspoon

- Coarse sea salt – 1 tablespoon

- Olive oil – 2 tablespoon

- 4 pound Bison chuck or beef – 1

- Garlic cloves (coarsely chopped) – 6

- Onion large (thinly sliced) – 1

- Red wine or water or chicken or beef stock water - 1 cup

Directions:

1. Smear the seasoning on the meat. Mix the vegetables in a small bowl. Leave out the roast covered with foil loosely for 1 to 2 hours at room temperature. You can also wrap it with foil and leave it overnight in a refrigerator.

2. Preheat the oven to 320 to 325 degrees Fahrenheit.

3. Take the olive oil in a large heavy casserole or Dutch oven and heat it (medium to high).

4. Brown the roast of all sides taking two minutes for each side and then set aside in a platter or plate.

5. Clean the pan of accumulated excess fat. Add wine, stock or water and scrap the pan so that it is de-glazed.

6. Place the roast in the pan again and put garlic and onions to cover it. Bake it for an hour.

7. Uncover the oven and continue roasting for another hour. For even cooking, stir the onions slightly and add more liquid (if required) after half an hour.

8. Put back the cover and continue cooking for one more hour. When the meat is fork tender, it is done.

9.   Remove the meat from the pot and keep it covered loosely with foil.

10. Strain the sauce and if required, season it with pepper and salt.

11. Slice the meat and separate the chunk, making it ready to serve.

Put some sauce on meat when serving.

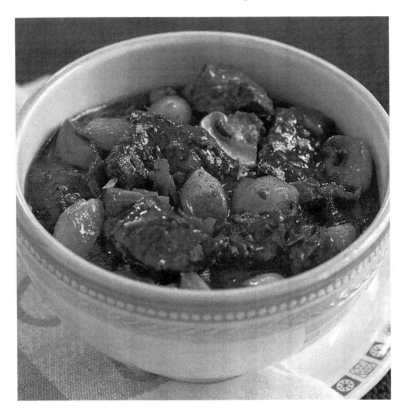

11. Beef Burgundy

Ingredients:

- Butter or lard – 4 tablespoons

- Bacon – ¼ pound

- Beef cubes (2 inches) cut from 2½ -3 pounds meat. Sirloin tip, chuck roast, rump roast and bottom or top are available options.

- Almond flour – 2 tablespoons

- Pepper – ¼ teaspoon

- Salt – 1 ½ teaspoons

- Carrots (sliced) – 2

- Tomato paste – 1 tablespoon

- Onion (sliced) – 1

- Garlic cloves (finely chopped) – 2

- Fresh parsley (finely chopped) – 1 tablespoon

- Fresh rhyme – 1 table spoon or 1 teaspoon if dried

- Brown or white crimini mushrooms – 1 lb.

- Beef stock – 2 ½ cups

- Bay leaf – 1

- Red wine (full bodied) – 3 cups

Directions:

1. Preheat oven to 425 degrees Fahrenheit.

2. Cut the bacon into short strips; take it in a deep saucepan and sauté with butter (1 tablespoon) till it is cooked but not crispy.

3. Use a paper towel to pat the beef dry and add it to bacon in 3 to 4 batches and brown every batch of meat before removing from pan.

4. Put the meat and bacon in the baking dish to be used in the oven and keep it aside.

5. Sprinkle almond flour, pepper and salt over the meat and bake it with the cover removed for 10 minutes so as to get the flour absorbed in the meat and creating a slight crust on the outside.

6. Take it out from the oven and lower the oven temperature to 325 degrees Fahrenheit.

7. Take the remaining fat from the meat and bacon in a saucepan and sauté it on the stove after adding butter (1 tablespoon) to it sauté the onion and carrots until it is soft. This may take about 8 minutes.

8. Add bay leaf, parsley, thyme, garlic and tomato paste.

9. Stir and add beef broth and wine and wait till it boils gently. Then set it to simmer for 3 to 5 minutes.

10. Now transfer the meat to the casserole pan and cook for 2 hours 30 minutes by covering the dish. The meat will become so tender that it can be easily pulled apart with fork, indicating that cooking is complete.

11. While the meat gets cooked, sauté the mushroom slices using the remaining butter. Avoiding crowding of mushrooms by doing it in 3-4 batches and set it aside.

12. When the meat is cooked, pour it in a colander with the liquid so that the liquid gets drained and is collected in a bowl placed under the colander.

13. Gently boil the liquid followed by 8 to 10 minutes of simmering.

14. Pour over the mushrooms and meat.

15. Before serving, garnish the dish with parsley.

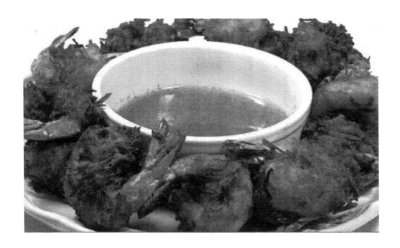

12. Garlic Coconut Shrimp

Ingredients (4 servings):

* Jumbo shrimp (frozen) – 20

* Coconut (shredded, unsweetened) – 2 cups

* Fresh garlic – as per your taste

* Coconut oil

Directions:

1. Add fresh garlic (grated) to coconut oil that you will have to melt in a bowl and toss shrimp so that it is completely covered.

2. Bread the shrimp on both sides with coconut flakes taken on a pan or plate.

3. Place it on baking sheet and bake for 20 minutes at 350 degrees Fahrenheit. The shrimp will turn pink to indicate that it is cooked.

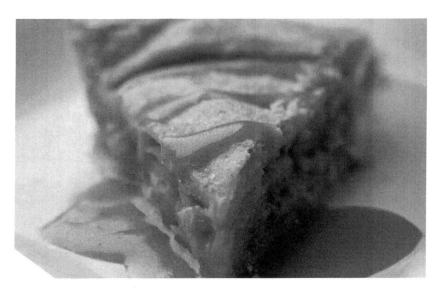

13. Cashew Cheesecake Pie (Raw Vegan)

The recipe consists of three parts – Cheese filling making, crumble crust and the rhubarb topping

Ingredients (2 servings):

*   Cashews – 2 cups

*   Agar powder – 1 tablespoon

- Water – 1 cup

- Coconut oil (melted) -3 tablespoon

- Agave nectar – 3 tablespoon

- Vanilla extract – 1 tablespoon or vanilla bean seed – ½

- Orange zest – 1 tablespoon (optional for flavoring)

- Almond extract – 1 teaspoon (optional for flavoring)

Directions:

1. Grind the cashews in batches in a coffee grinder in order to grind very fine.

2. Take water, cashews and agar agar in a bowl with your preferred flavorings, mix well and leave it overnight for complete soaking.

3. Next day, melt the coconut oil and agave and mix it.

4. Add this mixture to the cashew mixture and use a blender so that it mixes well. Adjust the sweetness to the level you desire by adding more agave or any other sweetener you prefer.

5. Spread the mix on top of your crumble crust and freeze it for a few hours so that it turns almost solid.

6. Put the rhubarb topping and savor the delicacy.

7. If you are using a heavy duty blender like Vitamix, soak the cashews in water overnight before grinding. The next day,

drain out the water and blend the cashews with agar powder and other ingredients.

8. Use Stevia if you want low calorie sweetener.

9. Next, make the crumble crust, assemble and put it in a freezer.

10. Make the rhubarb topping and put it on the cheesecake that is already frozen.

11. If you want you can take puree of frozen bananas or non dairy whipped cream in an icing bag and spread it like piping.

12. Best served frozen.

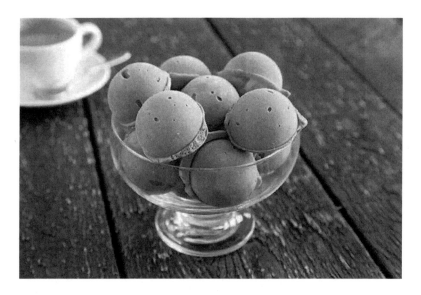

14. Bulletproof Fat Bombs

Ingredients (20 servings):

- Mascarpone cheese or creamed coconut milk

- or full fat cream cheese — 1 cup

- MCT oil – 2 tablespoon or additional coconut oil

- Grass-fed butter or extra virgin coconut oil – ¼ cup

- Brewed coffee (strong) or Dark Rum – ½ cup

- Stevia extract – 10 to 15 drops

- Cocoa powder (raw), unsweetened) – 2 tablespoons

- Swerve or Erythritol – ¼ cup

You can use 1 teaspoon rum extract instead of Dark Rum or Brewed Coffee.

Directions:

1. Take MCT oil, butter or coconut oil, cocoa powder and softened mascarpone in a blender.

2. Add Stevia or Erythritol and keep pulsing until smooth.

3. Pour lukewarm prepared coffee and pulse once more until smooth.

4. Transfer it to the ice-cream maker and process as instructed by the manufacturer of the equipment.

5. It may take half an hour to one hour depending on the ice-cream maker.

You can use a large ice tray of the size of 2 table spoons if you do not have an ice-cream maker.

Beverages Recipes

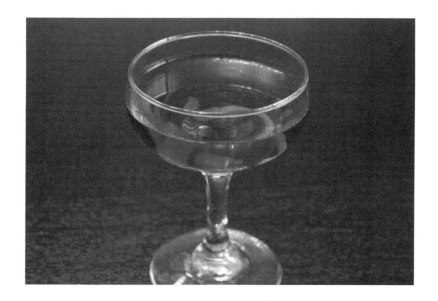

1. Bulletproof Manhattan Cocktail

Ingredients (single serving):

- Quality cherries in syrup jars or

- Amarena Italian cherries in 8oz jar – 1

- Bullet bourbon – 4 oz.

- Rosemary sprigs – 3

- Water – ½ cup

- Lemon juice – ½ oz.

- Ice

Directions:

1. Add ½ cup water to the cherry syrup that has to be poured in a small pot using a strainer.

2. Add rosemary to it by tossing, simmer for 2-3 minutes and remove from the heat so that the rosemary steeps into the cherry syrup as the mixture gets cooled thereby infusing flavor to it.

3. After cooling, put the cherries into the syrup again and leave it for 1 to 2 days in a refrigerator for chilling.

4. Mix ¼ cup (2oz) of the cherry syrup, lemon juice, ice and bourbon in a shaker and shake well so that the ice breaks into shards.

5. Pour the cocktail through a strainer into chilled martini glasses (two glasses).

6. Garnish the cocktail with a few cherries on 2 rosemary sprigs.

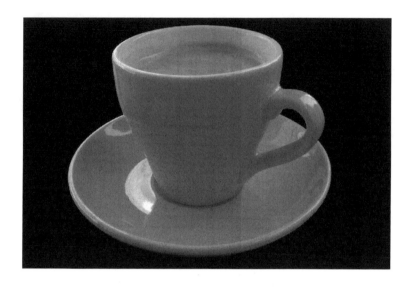

2. Bulletproof Coffee Knockoff

Ingredients (20 cups serving, serving size – 1 mug):

- Coconut oil – 1 ¼ cups

- KerryGold or Grass-fed butter or Grass-fed ghee – 8 oz.

- 20 big mugs of coffee – 1 at a time

- Heavy whipping cream – 20 oz. (optional)

- High quality cocoa powder – 1/3 cup (optional)

- Ez – Sweetz or your choicest sweetener – ¼ teaspoon

Directions:

1. Add coconut oil as per measurement in a deep bowl.

2. Add sweetener, cocoa powder and butter to coconut oil.

3. Use a microwave to melt the mixture in about half a minute (30 seconds) until it becomes very soft.

4. Blend the mixture in a blender. Use a high sided bowl if you are using an immersion blender.

5. Share the fat and chocolate mix in 20 containers (2oz each) and cover with the lids.

6. Put it in a refrigerator and cool to make it ready for use.

7. Transfer the contents of a container to your coffee cup so that it settles at the bottom.

8. Add ½ container heavy cream to your coffee.

9. Melt the mixture in a Microwave oven for 30 to 45 seconds.

10. Mix the fats with the cream using a wand like Aerolatte wand. You may use a blender to accomplish the task of slight whipping if you do not have a wand. Avoid formation of oil slick on cup top.

11. The coffee is now ready to be poured out for serving.

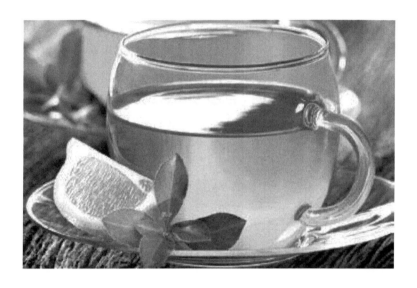

3. Bulletproof Green Tea

Ingredients (single serving):

- Matcha green tea or organic green tea – 1 glass

- Unsalted organic butter – 1 to 2 tablespoon (optional for vegans)

- MCT oil or coconut oil – 1 to 2 tablespoons

- Maca powder – 1 teaspoon (optional)

- Raw Cocoa powder – 1 tablespoon

- Pure vanilla extract – ¼ teaspoon

- Cinnamon – 1/8 to ¼ teaspoon or a few dashes

- Stevia (liquid) – 4 drops

- Sea salt – 1 pinch

- Vanilla protein powder – 1 to 2 teaspoon (optional for creamier taste)

Directions:

Mix all the ingredients in a blender. A hand blender will also do. Sip and enjoy.

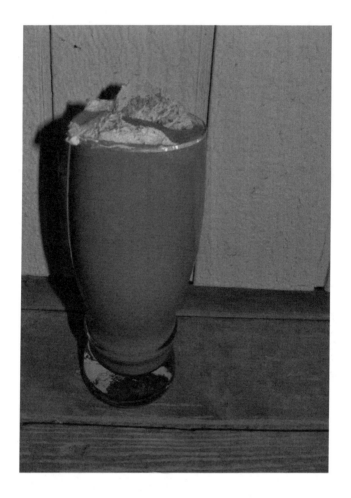

4. Bulletproof Matcha Tea Smoothie

Ingredients (single serving):

- Coconut oil – 1 teaspoon

- Vanilla almond milk (unsweetened) – 1 cup

- Spinach –

- Frozen banana – 1/2

- 2Matcha powder – 1 teaspoon (minimum)

- Protein powder (your favorite) – 1 scoop

Directions:

Do a perfect blending of the ingredients and enjoy.

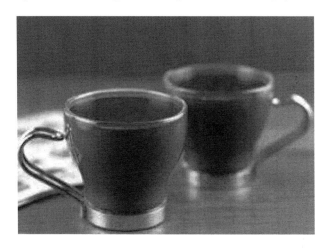

5. **Bulletproof Hot Cocoa**

Ingredients (single serving):

- Coconut milk (full fat) – ½ cup

- Unsalted grass-fed butter – 2 tablespoons

- Filtered water – ½ cup

- Cocoa powder (Raw or regular) – 2 tablespoons

- MCT oil or coconut oil – 1 tablespoon

- A dash of Cinnamon

- Vanilla extract – ¼ teaspoon

Directions:

1. Boil the coconut milk and water mix in a small sauce pan.

2. Mix all other ingredients with the boiling liquid in a mixing bowl (small).

3. Make it frothy by blending with a hand mixer or blender.

4. Pour it in a mug and enjoy.

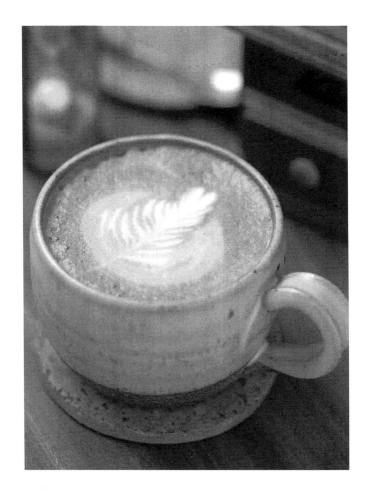

6. Bulletproof Latte

Ingredients (single serving):

- Hot coffee – 2 cups

- Coconut oil – 1 tablespoon

- Grass-fed butter – 2 tablespoons

- Cinnamon – 1 pinch

- Protein powder – 1 scoop

Directions:

Combine the ingredients in a blender and blend until frothy to get a velvety smooth delicious beverage.

SNACKS RECIPES

1. Bulletproof Chili –"Oh My Word"

Ingredients (4 servings):

- Grass-fed butter- 1 teaspoon

- Bulletproof upgraded XCT oil – 1 tablespoon

- Garlic cloves (chopped) – 4 to 5 (Keep aside an extra clove chopped

- Grass-fed ground beef – 1 ½ pounds

- Onions (chopped) – 1 cup (Keep aside an extra quarter cup)

- Chipotle chili powder - 1 teaspoon

- Ancho chili powder – 2 tablespoons

- Cummin (ground) – 2 tablespoons

- Organic tomatoes (medium, chopped) - 6

- Cayenne (red chili powder) - 1 teaspoon

- Water – 1 cup

- Basil (dried) - 2 teaspoons

- Fresh oregano (chopped) – 2 tablespoons

- Gluten-free beer – ½ cup

- Organic tomato paste – ¼ cup

- Organic chicken broth – ½ cup

- Cinnamon powder – ¼ teaspoon

- Bulletproof chocolate bar (grated) – ½ oz. (2 tablespoons approximately)

- Salt and pepper – according to taste

- Butternut squash (cubes tossed with upgraded XCT oil, salt and pepper) - 1

Directions:

Beef preparation

1. Heat butter and oil in a large skillet; add 4 chopped garlic cloves and ¾ cup chopped onions.

2. Sauté on medium heat till the onions become translucent.

Add beef, sauté until brown and use a spatula to break up the large pieces.

3. Add salt and pepper to beef to enhance taste.

4. When the beef turns brown, add cumin, red chili powder, chipotle and ancho and keep it aside.

Tomatoes preparation

1. Take the chopped tomatoes in a large kettle and add ¼ cup chopped onions, water, remaining quantity of chopped garlic clove and start simmering at medium heat for 4 to 5 minutes.

2. Add beer, cooked beef and chicken broth to the cooked tomatoes and set to simmer for another 2 to 3 minutes.

3. Add cinnamon and grated chocolate, stir it and start simmering for another 5 minutes. Then remove from heat and allow cooling.

Squash baking

1. Preheat oven to 350 degrees Fahrenheit.

2. Toss the butternut squash cubes with a tablespoon of Bulletproof upgraded XCT oil in a mixing bowl just to coat the cubes. Add slight salt, spread it on baking sheet and start baking until it becomes tender.

3. At the time of serving chili, heat it slightly and serve by adding baked butternut squash cubes.

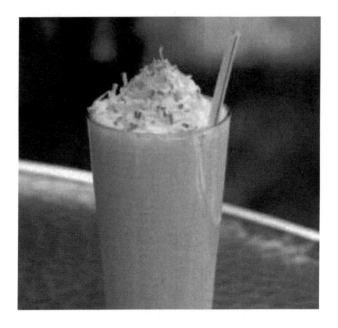

2. Bulletproof Coconut Smoothie

Ingredients (single serving):

- Bullet proof Brain Octane or MCT oil – 1 tablespoon (15 gram)

- Coconut milk (canned, full fat) – ½ cup

- Bulletproof Whey protein – 2 table spoons

- Mineral or filtered water – ¼ cup

- Vanilla bean

- Stevia (optional) for taste

- Lemon rind – ½ lemon (this is also optional)

Directions:

1. Mix MCT Oil or Brain Octane oil, coconut milk and vanilla in a milk frother or blender.

2. Add Whey protein; mix gently manually or at low speed in the blender to avoid the delicate Whey protein from being damaged.

3. The smoothie is ready to be served.

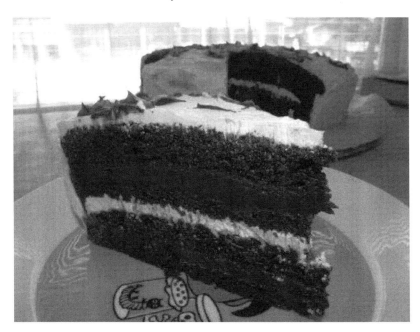

3. Dark Chocolate Mud Cake

Ingredients (serving of 10 to 12 pieces):

- Cocoa (sifted) – ½ cup (50 grams)

- Self raising flour (sifted) – 2/3 cups (100 grams)

- Sodi bicarb (sifted) – ½ teaspoon

- Plain flour (sifted) – 1 1/3 cups (200 grams)

- Double Espresso shot – 1

- 70% Cocoa Dark chocolate Pastilles – 250 grams

- Butter (unsalted, diced cubes of 1 cm) – 250 grams

- Extra large eggs (lightly beaten) – 4

- Caster sugar – 2 ½ cups (550 grams)

- Buttermilk – ½ cup

- Oil- 2 tablespoons (40 ml)

- Dark chocolate Couverture (chopped finely) – 200 grams

- Ganache

- Thickened cream – 200 ml

Directions:

Cake

1. Preheat oven to 160 degrees Fahrenheit. For fan forced oven it should be heated to 140 degrees Fahrenheit.

2. Grease lightly a 23cm round cake pan (deep) and line it with baking paper that extends above the pan by about 10 cm.

3. Mix the cocoa, flours and sodi bicarb in a large mixing bowl, stirring for good mixing.

4. Take coffee in a cup and add boiling water to bring the volume to 180 ml.

5. Take the coffee in a large sauce pan kept on vary low heat. Add chocolate, sugar and butter. Stir well for good mixing and continue it until butter and chocolate have melted to give a smooth mixture.

6. Set aside and allow it to cool a little. Add oil, milk and eggs to chocolate mixture. Keep whisking to ensure that it combines well.

7. Pour the chocolate mixture in the well that you will create at the centre of flour mixture and keep stirring until you are sure that it has combined well.

8. Pour the mixture in the cake pan that you have prepared, place it on a tray and put it n the oven to bake for 2 hours.

The clear emergence of a skewer from the centre indicates that baking is complete.

9. Remove the pan and place it outside for cooling, preferably on a wire rack.

Ganache

1. Heat cream in a sauce pan at low heat and remove it when it is just below boiling point.

2. Add chocolate while stirring gently. Leave it to stand for some time and then start gentle stirring. Continue the process until chocolate melts so as to give a smooth and shiny mixture.

3. Leave it to cool until it thickens enough to spread.

4. Apply to the sides and top of the cake with a spatula.

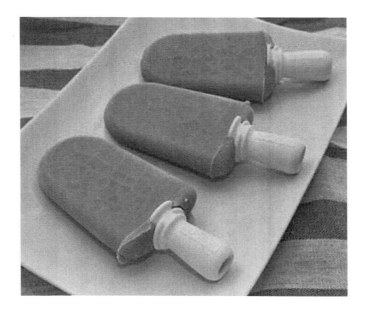

4. Bulletproof Coffee Strawberry Cream pops

Ingredients (single serving):

- Grass-fed unsalted butter – 1 tablespoon

- Egg white – 1

- MCT oil or coconut oil – 1 tablespoon

- Fresh strawberries – ½ cup

- Splenda – 1 packet

- Brewed cooled coffee- 1 cup

- Cocoa powder – 1 tablespoon

Directions:

1. Use a food processor to blend fresh strawberries until smooth. Add cocoa powder and cooled brewed coffee and set aside.

2. Make ready a cup of hot water to be used in double boiler.

3. Take the egg white with sweetener in a metal blow and place it in the double boiler.

4. Obtain a glossy, stiff and silky mass of the egg white mixture by beating it thoroughly.

5. Take the egg whites in a new bowl after taking out from double boiler. Add small butter pieces kept at room temperature. Before adding a piece ensure that the previous one has mixed completely. You get yellowish butter cream.

6. Add the cocoa, coffee, strawberry mixture and mix by whisking or using an electric mixer.

7. Pour the mass into Popsicle molds and leave it in a refrigerator for about an hour to allow its setting.

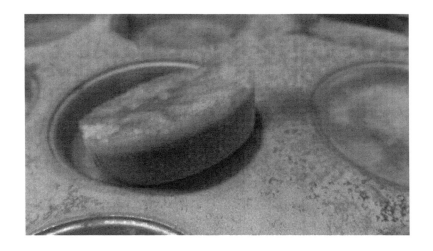

5. Bulletproof Coffee Pods

Ingredients (48Coffee Pods):

- Coconut oil – 1 ½ cups

- Butter – ¾ cup

- Doonks of Stevia – 3

- Vanilla – 1 ½ teaspoons

- Cocoa powder – 5 tablespoons

Directions:

1.   In a Microwave, melt coconut oil and butter in a glass measuring cup (1quart). Melting is to be done at intervals of

30 seconds with stirring between. Stir in vanilla, stevia and cocoa powder when the oil butter mix has fully melted.

2.   Fill two mini cup cake pans with the mixture, each pan having 24 cups.

3.   Solidify it by placing the pans in freezer.

4.   Pop out the pods with a knife when frozen and store them in a plastic bag in the refrigerator.

5.   Serve Bulletproof coffee with a coffee pod dropped into it. Enjoy its taste as it melts slowly into the coffee.

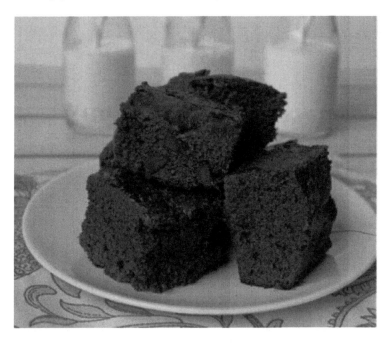

6. Bulletproof Low Carb Fudgy Brownies

Ingredients (16 brownies):

- Cocoa powder (unsweetened) – ½ cup

- Coconut oil (melted) – ½ cup

- Espresso powder – 2 teaspoons

- Sea salt – ¼ teaspoon

- Swerve – 1 to 1 ¼ cups (other granular sweetener may be used in powdered form)

- Vanilla extract – ½ teaspoon

- Liquid Stevia – ½ to 1 teaspoon

- Hazelnut flour – ¾ cup

- Eggs (large) – 3

- Cacao chocolate bar 70-90% (chopped) – 1.5 oz. (optional)

Directions:

1. Grease a square 8 inch baking pan and preheat oven to 350 degrees Fahrenheit.

2. Mix cocoa powder coconut oil, salt, espresso powder and powdered sweetener in a Microwave friendly large bowl and

Microwave for 1 to 1 ½ minutes, stirring at an interval of 30 seconds till the mixture becomes smooth and slightly heated. Alternatively, you can use a double boiler instead of Microwave.

3. Stir in vanilla and stevia. Add one egg at a time accompanied by brisk beating. Continue beating until batter is smooth and glossy. Stir in flour and blend evenly. Add chocolate chunks.

4. Using a rubber spatula, spread batter evenly in the pan that you have made ready and bake for 30 to 35 minutes. Do a tooth pick test to ascertain that baking is complete.

5. Remove from oven, wait for complete cooling and then cut it for serving.

DESSERT RECIPES

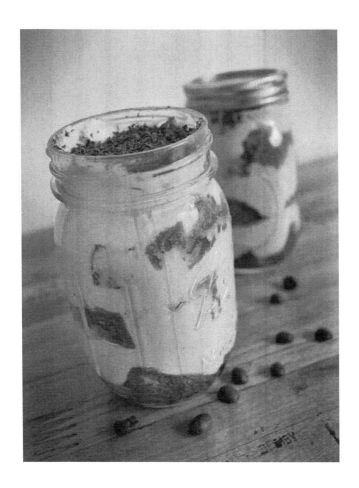

1. Bulletproof Tiramisu

Ingredients (6 servings):

- Xylitol – 2 tablespoons

- Organic eggs (separated)- 6

- Vanilla extract – 1 tablespoon

- Grass-fed butter (softened) – 50 grams

- Coconut flour – 1/3 cup

- Baking powder – ½ teaspoon

- Almond meal – 1/3 cup

- Soda bicarbonate – ½ teaspoon

- Salt – 1 pinch

- Upgraded Bulletproof coffee – 50 ml

- Pure cream – 125 ml

- Mascarpone cheese – 250 ml

- Kahlua – one dash (for flavoring)

- Liquid Stevia

- MCT oil – 1 cap full

Directions:

Sponge cake

1.   Preheat oven to 170 degrees Fahrenheit.

2. Make a cream of egg yolks, butter and xylitol in a mixer until fluffy and light. Leaving aside the egg whites, add all other ingredients and mix to combine well.

3. Whip egg whites in a clean bowl until soft peaks are formed.

4. Add 1/3rd of egg whites into the batter and repeat the process for two more times so that all ingredients get combined. The air from the egg whites should not be driven away.

5. Prepare a cake tin with proper greasing and place the batter in it. Bake for about half an hour to get a light spongy cake.

Tiramisu

1. Make a cup of Bulletproof Coffee and leave it aside to cool.

2. Completely whip pure cream and add Mascarpone cheese, 50 ml coffee. A dash of Kahlua, a cap full of MCT oil and a small amount of vanilla. Whip again till the mixture gets combined very well.

3. Make 1 cm slices of the sponge cake like fingers, dip the fingers into the coffee one by one and then layer the fingers with the cream mix.

4. You can use grated chocolate as topping and refrigerate it for a day for assimilation of the flavors.

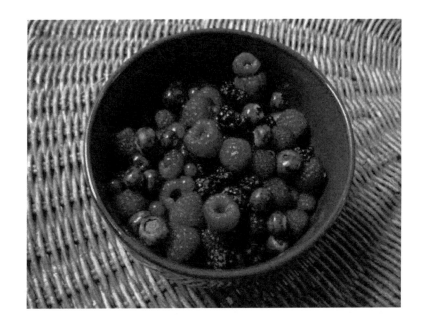

2. Berry Bowl

Ingredients (2 servings):

- Raspberries – ½ cup

- Blueberries– ½ cup

- Strawberries (chopped with stems removed) – ½ cup

- Fresh basil (chopped) – ¼ cup

- Lemon juice of half lemon

Directions:

Stir lemon juice and berries in a bowl. Use chopped basil as elegant topping.

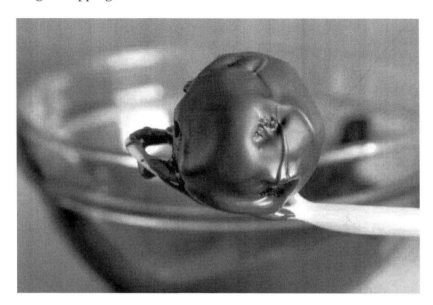

3. **Chocolate Truffle Pudding**

Ingredients (4 servings):

- Grass-fed gelatin – 1 tablespoon

- Coconut milk (full fat, divided, BPA free) – 4 cups

- Vanilla powder - 2 teaspoons

- Stevia or Xylitol – 4 tablespoons

- Grass-fed unsalted butter – 4 tablespoons

- Macadamia nuts and other garnish – ¼ cup (optional)

- MCT oil or coconut oil – 1 tablespoon

- Chocolate powder -3/4 cup

Directions:

1. Heat a cup of coconut milk, gelatin and xylitol over medium heat in a sauce pan until dissolved and then set aside.

2. Take the remaining coconut milk along with butter, vanilla; chocolate powder and oil blend thoroughly in a blender.

3. Add gelatin, hot coconut milk and nuts to a blender and mix it by pulsing.

4. Pour into ramekins or muffin tins and place it in a refrigerator for an hour to enable setting.

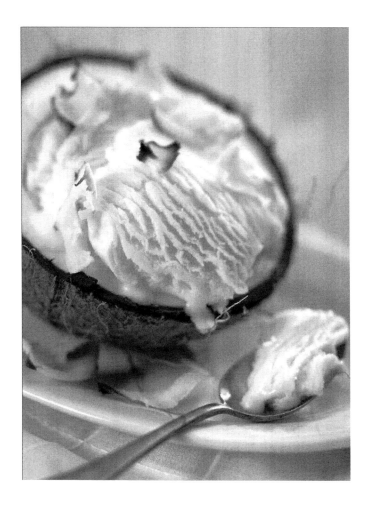

4. Coconut Ice Cream

Ingredients (4 servings):

- Egg yolks (pasteurized)- 4

- Whole pasteurized eggs - 4

- Ascorbic acid -1 gram or Apple cider Vinegar – 10 drops

- Vanilla powder -2 teaspoons

- Grass-fed unsalted butter – 7 tablespoons

- MCT oil - 3 tablespoons plus 2 teaspoons

- Coconut oil-7 tablespoons

- Chocolate powder – ¼ to ½ cup (optional)

- Ice or water – ½ cup

- Erythritol or Xylitol – 5 ½ teaspoons

Directions:

1. Add all the ingredients (except water or ice) in a blender and blend thoroughly to make the mixture creamy and soft.

2. Add half of ice or water to it and blend again to until you get a consistency like yogurt. For icier and firmer texture add more water.

3. Take the mixture in an in a cream maker and proceed as instructed by manufacturer.

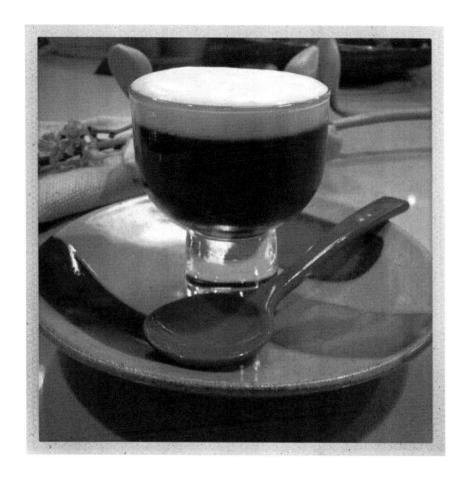

5. Bulletproof Coffee Jelly Dessert

Ingredients (single serving):

- Upgraded Coffee (freshly brewed) – 500 ml

- Upgraded Cocoa powder – 1 to 2 tablespoons

- Great Lakes unflavored gelatin - 3 tablespoons

- MCT oil – 20 to 30 grams (optional)

- Stevia sweet 90% powder – 1 knife tip

- Grass-fed unsalted butter – 50 grams

Directions:

1. Mix all the ingredients in a blender until combined well.

2. Take in a bowl and freeze it in refrigerator for 3 to 4 hours.

3. Served as it is with whipped cream.

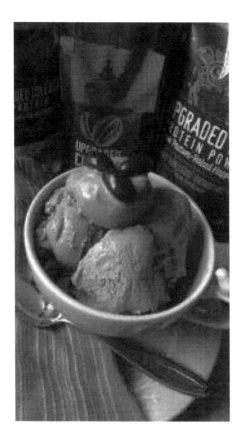

6. Bulletproof MoJoeJingLato

Ingredients (single serving):

*   Grass-fed ghee – 4 tablespoons

*   Upgraded Brain Octane oil or XCT oil (Bulletproof) – 2 tablespoons

- Upgraded Coffee (Bulletproof, freshly brewed) – 3 cups

- Upgraded Collage (Bulletproof) – 1 tablespoon

- Upgraded Cacao powder (Bulletproof) – 4 tablespoons

- Pearl powder - 2 teaspoons

- Non GMO Lecithin – 3 tablespoons

- Upgraded vanilla powder (Bulletproof) – 1 teaspoon

- Natural Xylitol (hardwood based) – 2 tablespoons or to suit your taste

- Ashwagandha – 1 teaspoon

- Eucommia bark – 1 teaspoon

- Upgraded Whey protein (Bulletproof) – 6 tablespoons

- Chocolate Stevia – 3 squirts or to suit your taste

- Vanilla Stevia - 4 squirts or to suit your taste

- Organic coconut milk – 1 cup

- Hazelnut Stevia - 4 squirts or to suit your taste

Directions:

1. Keep aside the whey protein, the liquid Stevia sweeteners and half cup coconut milk while taking all other ingredients in a blender and blend thoroughly.

2. Transfer the blended mixture into ice cube trays (non toxic) and put it in freezer.

3. After freezing, take the ice cubes into a blender (Vitamix gives best results) and add the whey protein, coconut milk and Stevia.

4. Use the plunger to smoothen the contents by pounding.

The Super Food is now ready for you.

Blending has to be done in two batches if you are not using a Vitamix.

Chapter 7

WRAPPING UP

Till now, a lot has been said about the bulletproof diets. We have discussed and learnt a lot regarding all the aspects of the bulletproof diet, that it is not only a mere diet but also the best lifestyle people can opt for. Those, who are going to follow a regular routine under Bulletproof diet, will definitely gain more energy and willpower than they have ever imagined. Few months in the bulletproof diet and you will surely experience the change!

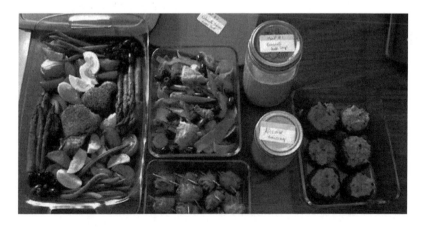

If you are suffering from high blood sugar, cholesterol, obesity and other related issues and health problems, start learning about the benefits of the bulletproof diet. Following a bulletproof diet along with the bulletproof excrcise will help you to reduce your health problems, while reducing weight. However, make sure you follow the diet sincerely, honestly and whole heartedly. The results will not be visible overnight. So, you need to be patient. The body and mind needs time to get adjusted with any of the new diet charts. Do remember that you have nothing to lose in the diet period; instead you are going to receive the utmost benefit.

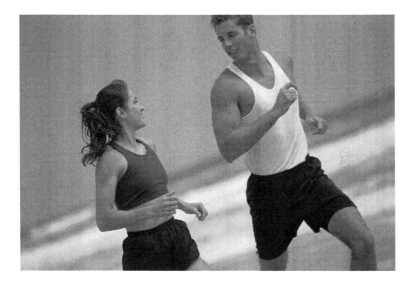

It is beyond any doubt that following the bulletproof diet routine throughout life will provide you optimum health. Just keep one thing in mind that before opting for the diet, do consult the doctor and be aware of the state of your health so that you can take precautions accordingly. The bulletproof diet will eventually teach you various methods to choose the proper food items. For starters, you need to go for food items with proteins, fats, and nutrients. Herbs and spices will make your meals even more delicious. So, are you ready to become bulletproof?

Thank you for reading! I really hope this book helped you in some way! If you'd like to check out my other books then click the link below!

http://www.amazon.com/Valerie-Childs/e/B00VVS8TYO/ref=ntt_athr_dp_pel_pop_1

At the link you'll find books on the Paleo Diet, Paleo Slow Cooker, Green Smoothie, Keto Diet, Mediterranean Diet, Dash Diet, Gardening and many more! Check it out!

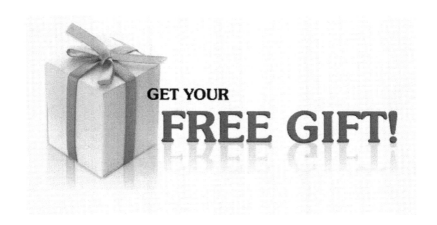

WAIT! – DO YOU LIKE FREE BOOKS?

My **FREE Gift** to You!! As a way to say **Thank You** for downloading my book, I'd like to offer you more **FREE BOOKS!** Each time we release a NEW book, we offer it first to a small number of people as a test - drive. Because of your commitment here in downloading my book, I'd love for you to be a part of this group. You can join easily here → http://smoothieslimdown.com/

Conclusion

Thank you again for downloading this book!

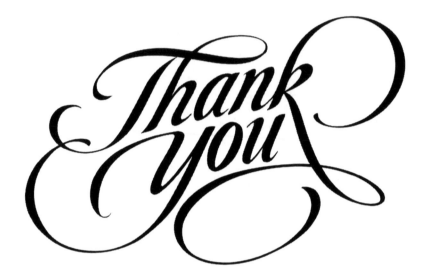

If you enjoyed this book, then I'd like to ask you for a favor, would you be kind enough to leave a review for this book on Amazon? It'd be greatly appreciated!

Help us better serve you by sending questions or comments to greatreadspublishing@gmail.com - Thank you!

Made in the USA
Middletown, DE
03 September 2015